BAILLIÈRE
SELF-ASSESSMENT

Revise General
Nursing
3

Christina Cheetham
SRN, RSCN, RCNT, Cert. Ed., RNT
Senior Tutor
Charles West School of Nursing
Great Ormond St, London

Joan Ramsay
SRN, DN(Lond.), Cert. Ed., RNT
Senior Tutor
Charles West School of Nursing
Great Ormond St, London

Baillière Tindall
London   Philadelphia   Toronto
Sydney   Tokyo

Baillière Tindall   24–28 Oval Road
W. B. Saunders   London NW1 7DX

                     The Curtis Center
                     Independence Square West
                     Philadelphia, PA 19106–3399, USA

                     55 Horner Avenue
                     Toronto, Ontario M8Z 4X6, Canada

                     Harcourt Brace Jovanovich Group (Australia) Pty Ltd.
                     30–52 Smidmore Street
                     Marrickville, NSW 2204, Australia

                     Harcourt Brace Jovanovich (Japan) Inc.
                     Ichibancho Central Building, 22–1 Ichibancho
                     Chiyoda-ku, Tokyo 102, Japan

© 1987 Baillière Tindall

First published 1987
Reprinted 1989 and 1991

Typeset by Photo-graphics
Printed in England by Clays Ltd, St Ives plc

British Library Cataloguing in Publication Data
Cheetham, Christina
    Revise general nursing 3.—
    (Baillière's self-assessment for nurses)
    1. Nursing—Problems, exercises, etc.
    1. Title II. Ramsay, Joan III. Series
    610.73'076 RT55

ISBN 0–7020–1198–3

Contents

Preface

The aim of this series of books is to provide the learner with an active means of independently evaluating his/her knowledge and understanding of patient care.

The books are intended for RGN students as a way of consolidating their previous knowledge. They could be used at the end of each unit of learning or as an aid to revision at the end of training.

It is probable that with the recent development of the state final examination, individual hospitals will have differing methods of assessment. However, whatever form of assessment is used, these books should provide a useful means for the learner to evaluate his/her own knowledge and understanding.

The three books are all sub-divided into five chapters, each concerned with a particular patient problem. The wide range of experience encountered by the learner during her training is covered within these chapters. Each chapter consists of a number of short case-histories and related questions.

The questions are concerned with the assessment, planning, implementation and evaluation of individual patients' care. The concepts of holistic nursing and research are seen as important aspects throughout. Suggested answers to questions are given after each case history.

Application of knowledge and problem-solving is seen as more important than recall of facts. This form of revision ensures that the learner understands the rationale for nursing care, and is able to be adaptable in different situations.

Acknowledgement must be made to the support and invaluable assistance given by Ms Richenda Milton-Thompson of Baillière Tindall.

Thanks also go to Mrs Susanne Walker and Mrs Maggie Wisby for typing the manuscript.

C. Cheetham

J. Ramsay

Introduction:
How to Use this Book

- This book has been designed to help you learn by yourself. You will find that it is divided into five chapters, each relating to a particular patient problem. Some you will have come across already; some you may meet later in your career. You might prefer to look at the problems you are familiar with first, as the sections do not inter-relate, and can be taken in any order.

- The book is primarily intended as a consolidation of your previous theoretical and practical experiences. Therefore, you may wish to do some preparatory reading or revision before you tackle any of the case-histories. You may also use them as a pre-test of your knowledge. You may know more than you think!

- Questions are worded differently. To help you decide the most appropriate way to answer each you may like to spend some time familiarizing yourself with the commonly used words as shown below:

  Define: to state precisely your meaning of
  Describe: to give an account or representation of, in your own words
  Discuss: to investigate, examine by argument (i.e. by logical discussion), to sift or debate ideas and to reach your conclusion
  Explain: to make plain, interpret or account for; to give the reasons for your actions
  Identify: to determine the individual characteristics of
  List: to give an item-by-item record
  Outline: to provide a draft account, giving the main reasons or general principles of a subject
  State: to present in a brief, concise format

- The style of your answers is entirely up to you. You do not have to write a timed essay; notes will do. However, we do suggest some kind of written response as educational research shows that this significantly improves memory. Any help in remembering must be worth using!

- Do not worry if your answers are slightly different to those given. Our answers are not intended to be the only correct ones, but do contain the essential points. Also, we realize that each hospital has its own local practices. You may have to adapt our answer to meet your own hospital procedure.
- You will find that some topics are very specialized. If you have not had experience in these specialities you may prefer to use such case-histories to extend your knowledge rather than as a basis for revision.
- You will also find that some questions in some case-histories relate to ward management and teaching junior colleagues. You may wish to omit these questions until you have had experience in these areas.
- We hope that you find this way of studying useful, and, most importantly, enjoyable! If so, you may be interested in the companion volumes to this book.

Other books by the same authors:

Revise General Nursing 1 covers the following topics:

- Care of the patient with problems of the heart and circulation
- Care of the patient with an endocrine disorder
- Care of the patient with problems of the alimentary and biliary tracts
- Care of the patient with a mental or physical handicap
- Care of the patient with problems of bones and joints

Revise General Nursing 2 covers the following topics:

- Care of the elderly patient
- Care of the patient with a sensory impairment
- Care of the female patient and her reproductive system
- Care of the patient with problems of the renal and urinary systems
- Care of the patient approaching death

Baillière's Nursing Study Aids *Crosswords for Revision*—30 crosswords to help students learn, covering the following topics:

Abdominal surgery; anaemia; ante-natal care; anorexia nervosa; asthma; cardiac failure; cerebrovascular accident; cholecystitis; chronic bronchitis; Crohn's disease; community care; diabetes mellitus; eczema; fractured femur; head injury; leukaemia; mastectomy; meningitis; myocardial infarction; nephrotic syndrome; non-accidental injury; paediatric gastroenteritis; peptic ulcer; psoriasis; pyloric stenosis; renal failure; rheumatoid arthritis; thyroidectomy; tonsillectomy; vaginal hysterectomy.

1 Care of the Patient with Respiratory Problems

1.1 John Reynolds—a young adult with asthma

You are in charge on night-duty when you are informed by the accident and emergency department that John Reynolds is to be admitted to the ward at 0200 hours with a severe attack of asthma. John is 19 years old and is a first year university student.

1   What preparations should the nurse-in-charge on night-duty make when the accident and emergency department informs her of John's impending arrival?

2   How should John's condition be explained to a junior nurse?

When John arrives on the ward he is sweaty, anxious and dyspnoeic. An intravenous infusion of 1 l normal saline containing aminophylline 500 mg and hydrocortisone 100 mg has been commenced in the accident and emergency department.

3   How may John's anxiety be controlled?

4   What percentage of oxygen should John be given? Why?

5   What is the significance of the observations the nurse should make on John during the rest of the night?

You notice while nursing John that he has eczematous lesions on his limbs. He has apparently suffered from eczema for some time but has never had an asthmatic attack before.

6   John is obviously embarrassed by the area of his red, inflamed skin. How can you reassure him?

After 5 days John is ready to be discharged. He has been prescribed sodium cromoglycate (Intal) via a spinhaler and a Salbutamol (Ventolin) Inhaler.

7 What advice should the nurse give John with regard to preventing further asthmatic attacks once he is discharged?

8 What advice can be given to John to help him avoid exacerbations of his eczema?

1.1 Answers

1 • John's bed should be situated where he can be observed easily and preferably near an open window.
  • Resuscitation equipment should be placed nearby (not obviously).
  • Oxygen cylinder and Ventimask should be on hand.
  • Any flowers and feather pillows should be removed.
  • Foam pillows should be arranged so that the patient can be placed in an orthopnoeic position.
  • An intravenous stand should be available.

2 Ask her to draw a bronchial tree to show the parts involved (to assess her present knowledge) (Fig. 1).

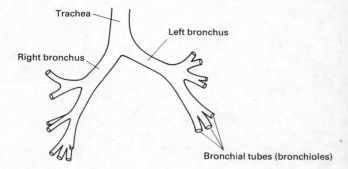

Fig. 1 The bronchial tree.

Explain that there is:
  • spasm of the smooth muscle of the bronchi and larger bronchioles
  • swelling of the mucosal lining
  • increased viscous bronchiole secretions

These changes all narrow the airways so that the inspiratory effort is increased. Wheezing on expiration occurs as air is forced out through the narrowed vessels.

These changes are due to an allergic response to:
  • dust, animal fur or similar allergens (extrinsic asthma)
  • psychological factors ⎫
  • respiratory infection ⎬ (intrinsic asthma)

3 Explain that this is an allergic condition (related to eczema) and although frightening will soon be controlled with the

drugs. You should also:
- stay with him
- ask only essential questions
- remain calm and confident
- help him to control his breathing pattern

4   John should be given 60–100% of oxygen. As this is his first attack of asthma he has no chronic obstruction of his airways, so his stimulus for breathing remains as a high arterial carbon dioxide level. He can be given a high percentage of oxygen to overcome his difficulty in inspiration without impairing his respiratory stimulus.

5

Observation	Significance
4-hourly temperature	• John is likely to be pyrexial, especially if infection is present. (Use the axilla while the patient is acutely breathless.)
1-hourly pulse and blood pressure	• Side-effects of the drugs used are tachycardia and hypotension.
1-hourly respirations	• Increased dyspnoea would indicate deterioration. • Pain on inspiration may indicate a pneumothorax. • Increased respiratory effort would also indicate deterioration.
Colour	• Cyanosis may indicate deterioration in condition.
Peak flow	• This may be used as a base-line to determine how the level improves after treatment.
Anxiety levels	• Restlessness may indicate deterioration or a side-effect of his drug treatment.
Sputum	• Yellow-green sputum indicates infection.

6   • Talk about his skin without showing distaste or embarrassment.
    • Do not be afraid to touch the lesions.
    • Neither stare at, nor ignore, the lesions.
    • Reassure him that his skin can be treated as well.

7

Advice about drug therapy
- 'Intal' is a preventative measure and should be taken regularly.
- 'Ventolin' is only to be used when John feels wheezy. It dilates the bronchioles. It should not be taken more than twice a day because it also increases the action of the heart.

Avoidance of allergens
- If the allergen is known, try to avoid it. Be wary of close contact with pets and very dusty/smoky atmospheres.
- Avoid infection wherever possible.
- Avoid stressful situations as far as possible.
- Teach stress reduction techniques, e.g. breathing exercises.

Promotion of health
- It is advisable not to smoke as cigarettes will irritate the affected area.
- Do not get overtired; this makes one more prone to infection.
- Encourage some form of sport, particularly swimming. (Sport provides a means of controlling breathing.)

8
- Avoid extremes of temperature.
- Use emollients in the bath to avoid dryness of skin.
- Use prescribed ointments sparingly.
- Avoid synthetic materials; these increase perspiration and make the lesions itch more.
- Avoid known allergens (see ans. 7).
- Avoid heavily perfumed toiletries.
- Try not to scratch lesions as this may lead to a secondary infection.

1.2 Mr Peacock—a man with chronic bronchitis

Mr Basil Peacock, aged 62 years, is a retired refuse collector. He has been admitted with an exacerbation of his long-standing chronic bronchitis and emphysema.

He is extremely dyspnoeic, cyanosed and expectorating copious amounts of purulent sputum. He is prescribed terbutaline 4-hourly via a nebulizer.

1 Explain the physiological changes that have led to Mr Peacock's problems.
2 Why is it important that Mr Peacock receives a particular percentage of oxygen?
3 What are the actual and potential problems to be considered in relation to Mr Peacock's oxygen therapy?
4 How may the above problems be overcome?
5 How may the nurse help Mr Peacock to expectorate?
6 Explain the significance of the observations to be made of Mr Peacock.
7 Mr Peacock has been prescribed terbutaline via a nebulizer. What are the actions and possible side-effects of this drug? How may the effectiveness of the drug be evaluated?
8 What advice should the nurse give Mr Peacock to help him to minimize his symptoms?

1.2   Answers

1
- **Dyspnoea** Constant irritation of the tracheo-bronchial tree suppresses normal cilial function. Thus, mucus and secretions are retained and form plugs in the smaller bronchi. Such plugs predispose to infection. Chronic infection destroys the pulmonary tissue, causing breathlessness.
- **Cyanosis** Progressive inflammatory changes lead to fibrosis and structural damage. The alveolar sacs become overdistended and their walls rupture, leading to destruction of the alveolar capillary bed. This results in poor gaseous exchange.
- **Copious sputum** Constant irritation of the tracheo-bronchial tree causes hypertrophy of the mucous glands and hypersecretion.
- **Purulent sputum** This results from infection.

2   The respiratory centre in the brain is usually sensitive to the level of carbon dioxide in the blood. If the carbon dioxide level rises, the respiratory rate and depth increase to breathe out this excess.

However, Mr Peacock will have a chronically high carbon dioxide level due to his chronic respiratory problem. In this situation the low level of oxygen in his blood becomes a respiratory regulator—the hypoxic drive to respiration. If Mr Peacock is given a high percentage of oxygen, this hypoxic drive will be lost and his respiratory rate will fall. This will eventually lead to further retention of carbon dioxide, apnoea and death (carbon dioxide narcosis).

Thus Mr Peacock should be given 24% oxygen via a Ventimask at no more than 2–3 l/min.

3   **Actual problems**
- Dryness of the mucous membranes of the eyes and mouth
- Difficulty in eating and drinking

Potential problems
- Danger of fire
- Mask is uncomfortable

4

Problem	Action
Dryness of the mucous membranes	• Provide 2–4 hourly mouth and eye care. • Encourage a 2–3 litre daily fluid intake. • Use humidified oxygen.

Difficulty in eating	• Provide easily digestible, small meals. • Make use of favourite soups and jellies.
Difficulty in drinking	• Use a flexible straw inserted through holes in a Ventimask. • Encourage favourite hot drinks to aid in loosening sputum.
Potential fire risk	• Warn the patient and visitors that oxygen is combustible. • Hang a 'No Smoking' sign.
Mask uncomfortable	• Place padding under the elastic and nose band if pressing on bony prominences. • Observe these areas for soreness.

5 • In conjunction with a physiotherapist inhalations should be encouraged to loosen secretions, followed by postural drainage and clapping.
 • Expectorants (such as Benylin) may be given as prescribed 4–6 hourly.
 • Hot drinks and humidified oxygen will also help to loosen secretions.
 • Deep breathing and coughing should be encouraged every 2–4 hours during the day.

6

Observation	Significance
Respirations	To note rate, depth and rhythm to monitor the effect of care and treatment. Increased dyspnoea would indicate a deterioration in his condition.
Sputum	To observe the presence of pus and infection indicated by yellow-green sputum. The amount should increase initially if expectoration is effective, then decrease as treatment lessens the amount of bronchial inflammation.
Pulse	Tachycardia may be a side-effect of terbutaline. Any arrhythmia may indicate heart failure.

Peak flow	Before and after drug therapy this will monitor Mr Peacock's response to treatment. As the bronchi dilate in response to treatment, the peak flow reading (forced expiratory volume in 1 second) should rise. The normal value is 400–500 litres.
Colour	Cyanosis should lessen in response to treatment.
Temperature	Pyrexia indicates infection, which should resolve with treatment.

7   Terbutaline is a bronchodilator. It acts on the sympathetic nervous system to relax smooth muscle and so dilate the bronchioles.

The possible side-effects relate to its action on other parts of the sympathetic system. It dilates blood vessels, which can cause tachycardia to a degree that causes the patient to experience palpitations and feel anxious.

Its effectiveness can be measured by estimating the patient's peak flow before and after taking the drug.

8   The nurse should advise Mr Peacock about the following:

- **Smoking** This should be avoided as it provides constant irritation to the respiratory tract and will further constrict the bronchioles. Smoky areas should be avoided for the same reasons.
- **Diet** A high protein and high vitamin C diet will help to protect against infection. A diet low in carbohydrates will prevent obesity, which makes breathing more difficult. Two to three litres of fluid per day will help to loosen secretions.
- **Warmth** Cold and damp should be avoided as these may precipitate infection. If the home is draughty, cracks, etc., should be plugged up with newspaper. The patient should sleep in a warm room with the window closed.
- **Breathing exercises** Mr Peacock should continue with the exercises taught by the physiotherapist to maximize lung function.
- **Features of infection** Increasing dyspnoea, fever and/or yellow-green sputum should be reported to his general practitioner.

1.3 Mr Pratt—an adult undergoing chest surgery

Mr James Pratt, aged 65 years, has been admitted to the ward for lobectomy. He was diagnosed as having carcinoma of the lung a fortnight ago and is aware of his diagnosis.

1 How should the nurse describe the proposed surgery to Mr Pratt?

2 How can the nurse ensure that Mr Pratt's respiratory function is at its optimum pre-operatively?

3 The night before surgery Mr Pratt says: 'This operation is a waste of time—I'm going to die anyway'. How might you react?

After his operation Mr Pratt returns to the ward with apical and basal underwater seal drains.

4 How can you explain to your junior colleagues the purpose of these drains?

5 What is the significance of the observations made in relation to his chest drains?

6 What precautions should the nurse take when caring for Mr Pratt's chest drains?

7 Respiratory insufficiency can be a complication of this type of surgery.
   (a) How can this be prevented?
   (b) How will the nurse recognize this?

8 How can the nurse explain to her junior nurse the reasons for Mr Pratt's physiotherapy?

1.3   Answers

1   Draw a simple diagram of the lungs (Fig. 2).

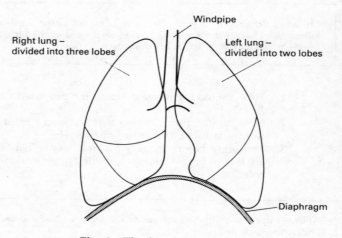

Fig. 2   The lungs.

Explain that the lungs are divided into segments or lobes. The surgeons are going to remove the diseased lobe of one lung without embarrassing respiratory function too severely.

Reassure him that removal of the part of one lung is quite compatible with life.

2   The nurse should:
● dissuade him from smoking.
● encourage physiotherapy (breathing exercises) to improve respiratory function as much as possible.
● observe any sputum for signs of infection (yellow-green in colour).
● record his respiratory rhythm and rate four hourly to assess any improvement.

3   It is important to recognize that this statement may be part of the depressive stage in the period following knowledge of a terminal illness. Ask Mr Pratt why he is saying this, giving him an opportunity to express his feelings. It may then be appropriate to ask the doctor to talk to him again about his forthcoming surgery.

4 During surgery, the opening of the chest causes atmospheric air to enter forcibly due to the negative pressure that normally exists in the thoracic cavity. This causes the lung to collapse. Therefore, after chest surgery the secretions and blood must be drained to allow the necessary re-expansion of the lung. Drainage must be by the closed (underwater) method to prevent the further entry of atmospheric air.

   • **The apical tube** drains air from the upper part of the cavity.
   • **The basal tube** drains blood and exudate from the base of the cavity.

5 The level of water should fluctuate ('swing') with each respiration. Failure to do so may mean that clogging of the catheter has occurred due to a blood clot or kinking. It can also mean that the lung has re-expanded.

   Check the colour and amount of the chest drainage. Bright red, copious drainage indicates haemorrhage. Measure any drainage to aid in monitoring the fluid balance.

6 The nurse should check that the drainage system is effective. The tube from the chest wall should always be under the level of the fluid in the drainage bottle. All connections should be airtight. The drainage bottle should be in a safe position on the floor. Ensure that all domestic and paramedical staff are aware that the drain must stay below the level of the patient's chest.

   • The nurse should also ensure that chest clamps are available to clamp off the chest tube as soon as any break in the system occurs.
   • The drainage bottle should *never* be lifted above chest level to prevent fluid flowing up the tube and into the pleural space. The tubes should be clamped if such movement is necessary when carrying out nursing care.
   • The drainage tubes should be milked *towards* the drainage bottle to prevent obstruction of the tubes by secretions.

7 (a) Respiratory insufficiency can be prevented by:
   • positioning the patient on his affected side to allow full expansion of the unoperated side.
   • monitoring his respiratory rate and rhythm and chest movements at least 4-hourly.
   • giving him continuous oxygen for at least 24 hours.
   • giving analgesia as prescribed on a regular basis to allow the patient to cooperate with coughing and deep breathing. Help by splinting the wound with the hands when the patient coughs.

- avoiding abdominal distension (with the help of a flatus tube, exercise and early ambulation) as this pushes up the diaphragm and hinders deep breathing.

(b) Respiratory insufficiency can be recognized by the following symptoms:

- cyanosis
- laboured, shallow respirations
- confusion (due to cerebral anoxia)
- a fast, irregular pulse

8   The reasons for Mr Pratt's physiotherapy are as follows:

- **Chest physiotherapy** Coughing and deep breathing aid in the removal of secretions and thus help to prevent lung collapse and chest infection.
- **Leg exercises** These improve venous return, which aids in the prevention of a deep vein thrombosis and a chest infection.
- **Posture and arm movements** These prevent deformity and stiffness of the affected side. The patient can exercise his arm on the affected side by raising himself upright by pulling on a rope attached to the foot of the bed.

1.4   Mrs Weston—a woman with pneumonia

Mrs Weston has been admitted as an emergency with a diagnosis of viral pneumonia. She fainted while at her early morning cleaning job.

Mrs Weston is 52 years old and looks after her husband, Percy, aged 63 years, who is confined to a wheel-chair with multiple sclerosis. She has been doing cleaning in the early mornings and evenings to enable her to look after her husband during the day.

On admission she is dyspnoeic, pyrexial and complaining of severe chest pain when she breathes in. She is also very anxious about her husband.

1   What immediate steps should be taken to look after Mr Weston?

2   How can the nurse relieve Mrs Weston's pleuritic pain?

3   How can the nurse relieve Mrs Weston's pyrexia?

4   Mrs Weston has been prescribed gentamicin 80 mg three times a day. What observations should be made to ensure that there are no adverse effects of this drug?

5   How can the nurse help to stimulate Mrs Weston's appetite?

6   What precautions should be taken to ensure that there is no spread of this infection?

7   Mrs Weston continues to worry about her husband. How can she be reassured?

8   How can Mr and Mrs Weston's situation be helped when Mrs Weston is ready to go home?

1.4   Answers

1   • A police message will ensure that Mr Weston is safe for the immediate time.
   • The Westons' general practitioner will contact the community nurse, who will assess Mr Weston's needs, and the social services, who will provide help as necessary.

2   • Encourage Mrs Weston to cough, splinting the painful area.
   • Position the patient on the side of the pain (This helps to splint the painful area and allow full expansion of the other side of the chest.)
   • A heating pad should be applied.
   • Offer aspirin 300–600 mg 4–6 hourly as prescribed.

3   The following should be made available:
   • tepid sponges (if she has hyperpyrexia)
   • a fan
   • a bed-cradle to allow movement of air
   • cotton nightclothes (to be changed when wet with perspiration)
   • minimal bedclothes
   The nurse should do the following to relieve Mrs Weston's pain:
   • sponge Mrs Weston's face and hands.
   • Encourage her to drink cool fluids.
   • Take her temperature via the axilla. (Coughing and mouth breathing will make the oral method inaccurate.)
   • Offer her aspirin (as above).

4   Record the urinary output and report any poor output(less than intake by 10% or more) as gentamicin is nephrotoxic.
   Note any dizziness, complaints of hearing loss, or ringing in the ears as gentamicin is also ototoxic and has been known to damage the vestibular or auditory branch of the eighth cranial nerve.
   (Blood levels will be taken on alternate days to monitor the levels of the drug circulating in the body.)

5   • Offer her only small quantities of food.
   • Find out her likes and dislikes.
   • Give her a soft diet so that eating does not further embarrass breathing.
   • Ensure that her mouth is clean.

6   • Mrs Weston's bed should be placed in a well-ventilated part of the ward.
   • Mrs Weston should not be positioned near those patients

particularly at risk to infection, e.g. the elderly, post-operative patients, patients with chronic chest conditions, patients who are immunosuppressed.

- Remind the patient to cover her mouth when coughing, and keep the lid on the sputum pot.
- Sputum pot and tissues should be changed at least twice a day. Used materials should be incinerated.
- Wash your hands after attending to Mrs Weston.

7
- Arrange a visit from her husband.
- Arrange daily telephone calls.
- Ask her friends/neighbours to visit and to report on Mr Weston's progress.

8
- Involve Mrs Weston and assess the present situation.
- Consult the medical social worker—Mrs Weston may be entitled to supplementary benefits.
- Mrs Weston should consider taking early retirement.
- Community nursing staff should help Mrs Weston to care for her husband.
- Mr and Mrs Weston should be put in touch with the Multiple Sclerosis Society to meet and talk to others in the same situation.

1.5   Mr Morris—a young man who has had a pneumothorax

Michael Morris, aged 22 years, is a physical education teacher. After playing rugby he experienced severe chest pain. His friends thought he was having a heart attack and took him to hospital. In the accident and emergency department a pneumothorax was diagnosed and a chest drain was inserted.

Michael was then transferred to the ward.

1   Now that Michael is more comfortable he asks you to explain his condition. How can you explain a spontaneous pneumothorax?

2   What fluid is put into Michael's drainage bottle? Why is this particular fluid chosen?

3   Which is more important and why:
   (a) to have a standard amount of fluid in the drainage bottle?
   (b) to have enough fluid to cover the end of the tube leading from the chest?

4   Construct a problem-solving care plan for Michael for the first 24 hours following the insertion of his chest drain.

Three days later while you are in charge of the ward a junior nurse slips on a patch of wet floor, twisting her ankle and breaking Michael's chest drain.

5   As the nurse in charge of the ward, select 10 of the following actions, giving reasons, and place them in order of priority to deal with this situation. (Actions to be carried out simultaneously should be bracketed together.)

Possible actions
- Arrange for a chest X-ray.
- Lie Michael flat.
- Inform the nursing office.
- Take and record half-hourly pulse and respirations.
- Delegate a senior nurse to stay with Michael.

- Prepare and connect another drainage bottle.
- Inform the houseman.
- Clamp the chest drain.
- Reassure Michael.
- Reassure the injured nurse.
- Delegate someone to care for the injured nurse.
- Investigate why the floor was wet.
- Ensure that the broken glass is cleared away.
- Ensure that the wet floor is mopped dry.
- Order a porter to take the injured nurse to the accident and emergency department.
- Record the incident.
- Encourage Michael to cough.
- Observe Michael's colour and administer oxygen if cyanosis is present.

6 On the fifth day following his admission the water in Michael's chest drain stops fluctuating. List all the reasons for this occurrence. How can it be determined whether this means that the affected lung has re-expanded?

7 Giving reasons, describe the procedure for the removal of Michael's chest drain.

8 Before discharge Michael asks if his job puts him at risk of further pneumothorax. How should the nurse reply?

1.5   Answers

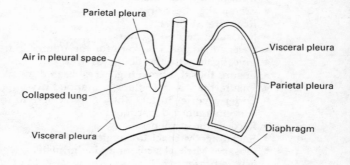

Fig. 3   Pneumothorax of the left lung.

1   Show Michael the above diagram. Show the normal anterior and posterior views on the right side and explain that 'pneumothorax' means that there is a collection of air in the pleural space (on the left side in Fig. 3) which has caused the left lung to collapse. Explain that normally the pleural cavity is only a potential space.

In Michael's case (a spontaneous pneumothorax) the air has entered the pleural space due to a ruptured air-sac on the surface of the visceral pleura. It is not known why this occurs but it is fairly common in young, healthy, active men.

This rupture will heal over and the air in the pleural cavity will be gradually absorbed, allowing the lungs to expand. The chest drain will create a vacuum to prevent inhaled air from escaping from the lung while the ruptured area is healing.

2   Sterile water or sterile normal saline will be used in Michael's drainage bottle as these fluids are less hazardous should any incident occur where the fluid is allowed to enter the pleural cavity (e.g. where the drainage bottle is lifted above the level of the patient's chest).

3   (b). It is *most* important to have enough fluid to cover the end of the chest tube or the apparatus will be ineffective as no vacuum will be created.

4

Problem	Aim	Nursing care	Evaluation
Anxiety	To enable Michael to relax	• Explain the chest drain and related procedures. • Show Michael how to move around in bed without fear of dislodging the drain.	Michael appears relaxed and able to rest.
Pain at site of drain	To make Michael comfortable and willing to deep-breathe and cough	• Handle the drain site only when necessary. • Give analgesia, e.g. dihydrocodeine 25 mg, before physiotherapy and 4–6 hourly as required. • Pin the tubing to the bed to allow Michael free movement without pulling on the tube.	Michael says that he is comfortable and able to cooperate with physiotherapy.
Potential secondary pneumo-thorax (due to breaking of vacuum system)	To keep the drainage system intact	• Keep two large artery forceps by the bedside to double-clamp the tubing when changing the bottle. • Check that the bottle is positioned flat on a firm surface.	The water is fluctuating in the tubing.

		• Reinforce the connections with waterproof tape. • When transporting the patient, carry the bottle in a holder. • Check for fluctuation of water in the tubing.	
Potential obstruction of tubing	To keep the tubing patent	• Ensure that the tubing is not kinked. • Ensure that the bottles are kept below the level of the bed (unless the tubing is clamped). • Milk the tubing as necessary.	The water is fluctuating in the tubing.
Potential infection from drainage system	To prevent ascending infection via the equipment	• Wash hands before handling the drain site or changing bottles. Check the drain site for inflammation. • When disconnecting the bottle, cover the end of the tubing with sterile gauze. • Take 4-hourly temperature readings to observe for pyrexia.	There are no signs of infection (pyrexia, redness of drain site).

| Potential tension pneumo-thorax | To prevent tension building up within the thorax | • Never clamp the tubing unless changing the bottle.
 • Observe Michael for dyspnoea, chest pain and shock. | Michael shows no signs of tension pneumothorax. |
| Loss of in-dependence | To help Michael with the activities of daily living | • Help with hygiene needs.
 • Help Michael to sit out of bed and mobilize gently. | Michael is able to manage most activities with help. |

5

Priority	Action	Reason
1	Clamp tubes.	To prevent air from escaping from the chest and to prevent collapse of the lung
2	Reassure Michael.	To gain his trust and cooperation
3	Observe Michael for cyanosis and administer oxygen if necessary	To prevent respiratory distress
4	Sit Michael up.	To enable him to breathe more easily
5	Delegate a senior nurse to stay with Michael.	To enable her to observe for signs of pneumothorax
6	Reassure the injured nurse.	To allay any feelings of guilt.
7	Delegate someone to care for the injured nurse.	To accompany her to casualty.
8	Prepare and connect another drainage system.	To reconnect the underwater seal drainage system
9	Ensure the broken glass is cleared up.	To prevent further incidents
10	Ensure that the floor is mopped up.	To prevent further incidents

These are your 10 priorities. Other actions (e.g. recording

the incident, investigating why the floor was wet) also need to be done but not immediately.

6 The fluctuation may cease if:
- the chest tube is kinked, looped or wedged under the patient
- the chest clamps have been inadvertently left on
- the chest tube is blocked
- the lung has re-expanded

You can determine whether the lung has re-expanded by checking the first three reasons listed above. If a blockage is suspected ask your patient to cough. If this produces no fluctuation of the water, the lung has probably re-expanded. This will be confirmed by a chest X-ray.

7

Action	Rationale
The chest tube is clamped for 24 hours.	To determine whether this causes any discomfort (i.e. whether the lung is not fully re-expanded)
The doctor orders a chest X-ray.	To check for re-expansion
The procedure is explained to the patient and analgesia is given 1 hour before removal.	To gain the patient's cooperation
Using an aseptic technique: • prepare a dressing trolley with the necessary equipment • remove any dressing around the chest tube and the suture securing it	To prevent infection from entering the thoracic cavity
The patient is instructed to inhale deeply and hold his breath while the tube is quickly removed in a gentle, controlled manner.	To prevent air from being sucked into the patient's chest

As the tube is removed the purse-string suture around the chest wound is pulled tight.	To prevent escape of air
The wound site is quickly covered with vaseline gauze and strapping.	To prevent escape of air

8 You should reply that it is sometimes possible for individuals to have repeated episodes of spontaneous pneumothorax but that he should not give up his job on this possibility alone.

Surgery is possible (pleurodesis or pleurodectomy) for recurrent pneumothorax. His job does not put him at any special risk of recurrences.

1.6 Mrs Khan—a woman with tuberculosis

Mrs Khan is a 38-year-old Indian woman who came to this country with her husband 20 years ago.

Mr and Mrs Khan own a small grocery shop and live above the shop with their four small children and Mr Khan's parents. Mrs Khan was admitted to the hospital with suspected pulmonary tuberculosis, following a history of weight loss, pyrexia and cough. She speaks very little English and is obviously scared of the ward environment.

1 What are the likely reasons for treating Mrs Khan in hospital rather than at home?
2 Mrs Khan is unable to expectorate sputum. Explain how the necessary specimens may be obtained.
3 What observations would be made to ensure Mrs Khan is not developing any side-effects to her chemotherapy?
4 Identify the precautions that should be taken to ensure that there is no spread of Mrs Khan's infection.
5 Describe the responsibilities of the occupational health department with regard to the protection of hospital personnel involved in the care of Mrs Khan.
6 Describe how the spread of Mrs Khan's infection into the community can be prevented.
7 What is the Mantoux test? How can a positive result be recognized?
8 How can Mrs Khan's problems with communication be helped?
9 What advice must be given to Mrs Khan (via her interpreter) before she is discharged?

1.6 Answers

1 Admission to hospital depends on the following:
- **the degree of illness** If the disease is at an advanced stage, rest in hospital may be advisable.
- **the patient's living conditions** If Mrs Khan is living in a crowded environment, others may be better protected by her admission to hospital.
- **socioeconomic or psychological problems** These may deter from effective treatment (i.e. rest) at home.
- **compliance of the patient** Mrs Khan speaks little English and may not fully understand the need for continuous treatment.
- **young children in the family** Mrs Khan may infect them.
- **occupation** Mrs Khan's job involves handling food.

2 By gastric aspiration—tubercle bacilli reach the stomach from the lungs when sputum is raised but swallowed rather than expectorated. Mrs Khan will be given nothing by mouth overnight. A nasogastric tube will be passed in the morning before food or liquid has been taken. A specimen of gastric contents can then be aspirated.

3

Drug	Possible side-effects	Observation
Isoniazid	Peripheral neuritis, hepatitis	Pins and needles in toes and fingers, and jaundice
Streptomycin	Damage to the auditory nerve	Gross hearing loss, vertigo or tinnitus
Rifampicin	Liver dysfunction (rare) discolours urine pink.	Jaundice Reassure Mrs Khan if her urine is pink.

In general, isoniazid, streptomycin, para-aminosalicylic acid, ethambutol and rifampicin are the most effective drugs used in the treatment of tuberculosis.

Isoniazid is considered the basic drug and is given in combination with one or two others depending on the activity and extent of the disease and physician's preference.

4 Mrs Khan should be nursed in a well-ventilated single room. Staff should wash their hands after caring for Mrs Khan. Mrs Khan should be advised to cover her mouth and dispose of tissues in a disposal bag which should be sent for inciner-

ation. There is no need for barrier nursing as chemotherapy is rapidly followed by reduction and elimination of the bacilli; also isoniazid is excreted in the sputum to act on expectorated bacilli.

5   All staff who have been involved in Mrs Khan's care should have a normal chest X-ray, and either a positive Mantoux test or a BCG immunization.

6   The health visitor (contact tracing) is responsible for searching out Mrs Khan's close contacts outside the immediate family.

Mrs Khan's children should be given isoniazid. (If their Mantoux test is negative in 3 months this can be discontinued.)

Her husband, parents-in-law and any other close contacts should be given a Mantoux test. If this is negative, isoniazid should be given and a chest X-ray taken to exclude active disease.

7   **The Mantoux test** An intracutaneous injection of either old tuberculin or a purified protein derivative from the tubercle bacilli; interpretations of the test are made after 48 hours. The area of induration indicates how positive the test is. A positive result (10 mm diameter induration or more) means that infection with tubercle bacilli has occurred previously and that antibodies to the tubercle bacillus are present.

8   Contact an interpreter via the medical social worker. With the help of the interpreter find some essential words to use and make use of picture cards.

Do not hurry or shout at Mrs Khan. Make full use of sign language to convey your meaning.

If any of Mrs Khan's family can speak English well, try to sort out problems when they are available. Try to explain any procedure with them to allay Mrs Khan's anxieties and try to arrange that they can be present.

9   Mrs Khan must take her drugs as prescribed uninterruptedly to prevent the infecting organism from becoming drug resistant.

She should prevent contamination of the air with the infecting organism (and thus the possibility of infecting others) by:

- covering the nose and mouth when coughing, sneezing or laughing
- placing used tissues in a paper bag which should be burnt
- avoiding kissing her family on the mouth

2 Care of the Highly Dependent Patient

2.1   Mrs Brown—a young woman with severe burns

Karen Brown, aged 26 years, has been admitted to the accident and emergency department following a cooking accident. A pan of fat caught fire and she has sustained partial-thickness burns to the face, hands, neck, right arm and chest. She is brought in by ambulance accompanied by her husband, who is obviously very distressed.

1   Describe the first aid of burns in an incident such as this.
2   How should the nurse assess the severity of Karen's condition when she arrives in the department?
3   What are the priorities of Karen's care when she first arrives in the accident and emergency department?
4   How would you explain to a junior colleague the significance of partial-thickness burns?

After initial care in the accident and emergency department, Karen is transferred to the intensive care unit. She is placed in a warmed (24°C) side room. Her facial burns are cleaned with saline and a bactericidal cream is applied. The other areas are covered with Bactigras after cleansing. Her hands are enclosed in boxing glove dressings and elevated.

5   Explain why Karen is particularly at risk of respiratory distress. How can this potential problem be managed?
6   Outline the prevention of infection of Karen's burns.
7   Describe the significance of Karen's observations for her first 72 hours in the unit.
8   How should Karen's nutritional needs be met?
9   What care should be planned to prevent Karen from developing contractures of her burnt areas?
10   Describe the psychological care that Karen and her husband will require.

2.1 Answers

1
- An ambulance should be called urgently since an early assessment of a burn and prompt medical intervention can minimize the development of complications.
- If the clothes are alight the patient should be laid on the ground and a blanket, rug or coat can be used to smother the flames.
- If the room is filled with smoke the victim should be taken outside as a priority; smoke inhalation can be a cause of death by itself.
- Any clothing that is not adhering to the skin should be removed.
- Continuous dousing of the burnt area with cold water will relieve pain and reduce the depth of the burn if performed soon after the incident. The eyes should be rinsed in large amounts of clean, cold water.
- Rings, bracelets and wrist-watches should be removed before oedema develops and causes constriction.
- The patient should be reassured constantly to minimize shock.
- The patient should not be given anything to eat or drink.

2 In order to assess the severity of Karen's burns the following should be considered:
- **The size of the burn injury** Using the 'rule of nines' (see Fig. 4) Karen's burns involve about 25% of her total body surface.
- **Depth of burn** This can be assessed by inspection of the burnt area. Partial-thickness burns appear red and large. Thick-walled blisters will be present.

  Karen will be in pain, unlike the patient with full-thickness burns whose skin will be anaesthetized to pain and temperature.
- **The part of the body involved** Burns of the neck and chest can hamper respiration. Burns of the hands and face require long-term intensive care and thus carry a poor prognosis.

  Karen should be observed for any difficulties with respiration due to the constrictive contraction of the skin on her neck or chest, or due to injury to the respiratory tree caused by smoke inhalation. Respiratory injury can also be identified by noting singed nasal hairs or carbon particles in the mouth, nose or sputum. Blood gases and a chest X-ray will aid the diagnosis of inhalation injury.

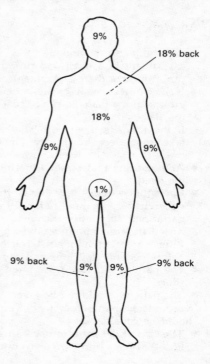

Fig. 4 The 'rule of nines' for assessing the size of burn injury.

- **The cause of the burn** Burns caused by flame or hot fat, such as Karen's burns, are known as thermal burns. Because they are dry burns, burnt areas can be much deeper and more serious than they appear.
- **Karen's age and general health** Karen is young and should be less susceptible to infection than the very young or the very old.

  Resistance to infection and stress also depends on her general health. You should check with her husband that she has no medical history (e.g. diabetes, asthma, steroid therapy) which would further complicate matters.

3

1 **To maintain an airway** Karen's head should be extended over a rolled towel. Suction should be readily available. Close observation should be made for dyspnoea and depressed chest movements as intubation may be necessary.

2 **To provide pain relief** Pain will add to Karen's shock and should be relieved as a priority. Morphine (or its derivatives) should not be used in this situation as it depresses respiration.

Reassurance and a competent approach will also help to allay shock.

3 **To prevent infection** Karen's clothing will be gently removed, cutting them if necessary. Wounds will be lightly covered with sterile cotton cloths. Intramuscular tetanus toxoid or immunoglobulin will be given. Hair may need to be shaved on and around burns of the head.

4 **To prevent hypovolaemic shock** An intravenous infusion will be commenced and human plasma protein fraction or dextran 110 in saline infused. The correct rate is best controlled by a mechanical drip counter. Half-hourly observations of Karen's pulse and blood pressure will be recorded as tachycardia and hypotension may indicate that the infusion is not combating shock. A central venous pressure line will also allow cardiovascular monitoring and will allow fluids to be replaced quickly.

Hypovolaemic shock can also be monitored by measuring Karen's urine output hourly. A self-retaining catheter will be passed to facilitate this. An output of less than 30 ml per hour should be reported as acute renal failure can be a complication of hypovolaemia.

4   To assess your junior colleague's present knowledge, ask her to draw a diagram of the skin. You can then shade in the affected area in a partial-thickness burn. The junior nurse can then be involved by identifying the function of each part of the skin damaged in the burn (see Fig. 5).

You can then explain the significance of the partial-thickness burn by explaining how the functions of the skin are affected. The main function of the skin is to protect the body from infection. In a burn the bacterial barrier is destroyed. Overwhelming infection is often the cause of death in a burns patient.

Other functions of the skin that may be affected are as follows:
- The skin normally controls fluid loss from the body by its waterproof epidermis. Damage to the epidermis in a

burn contributes to fluid and electrolyte loss by allowing evaporation.

- Damaged skin can no longer regulate body temperature. Uncontrolled evaporation by radiation, conduction and convection results in a massive heat and energy loss.
- Partial-thickness burns destroy part of the dermis. As long as some dermal cells remain the area can regenerate. Deeper partial-thickness burns which destroy all the dermis will require skin grafting.

The nursing care of a burns patient must take into account these changes to the function of the skin. Karen must be isolated in a cubicle and reverse-barrier nursed to prevent infection. The cubicle should be heated to about 25°C to maintain the correct body temperature. A careful account of fluid balance must be kept to monitor the fluid and electrolytes lost.

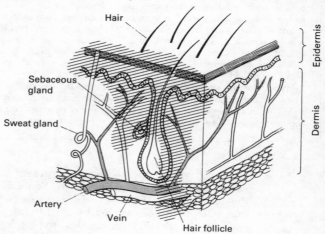

Fig. 5 Structure of the skin with shading indicating area affected in a partial-thickness burn.

5   Karen may have inhaled hot air, smoke or noxious chemicals if her accident occurred in an enclosed space. Inhalation of these substances causes direct damage to the respiratory tract. An inflammatory exudate is produced which prevents gaseous exchange. It also renders the patient more susceptible to chest infection.

As oedema develops, any circumferential burns of the neck and chest will contract and will thus constrict movements of the chest.

Management in the intensive care unit
- Karen will be nursed upright, supported by pillows.
- If exudate is present suction will be necessary at least hourly. (A tracheostomy may be performed to maintain the airway and facilitate suction.)
- Chest physiotherapy should be performed 4-hourly to encourage Karen to expectorate exudate. Two-hourly change of position, postural drainage and deep breathing exercises may help to loosen secretions. Nebulized mucolytics may also be given.
- Four-hourly monitoring of blood gases will indicate if artificial ventilation is required.

The nurse should observe Karen for tachycardia, dyspnoea, wheezing and restlessness, which will indicate inadequate oxygenation and the need for artificial ventilation.

Escharectomy—the surgical removal of thick, tenacious scabs—may be performed on any full-thickness burns that are hindering chest movements.

6
- Karen should be given protective isolation in a cubicle. All personnel and visitors entering the room should wear gown, gloves and mask.
- The introduction of infection should be avoided. Nasal and throat swabs should be taken from Karen on admission to ensure that her own flora do not contaminate the burns.
- Swabs must also be taken from the nursing staff. Any nurses with haemolytic streptococci will not be allowed to care for Karen.

   Equipment should not be borrowed from other patients for Karen's use. Ideally she should have her own equipment. If this is not possible it should be cleaned with an antiseptic before being placed in the cubicle.
- The burn wounds should be treated with a non-touch technique. If hands must be used, sterile gloves should be worn.
- Karen should be observed for signs of infection. This is best done by the appearance of the burn wounds. Any discharge or smell of the wounds should be reported. Swabs should be taken for microscopy, culture and sensitivity on alternate days.

> • Systemic antibiotics (e.g. penicillin or gentamicin) may
>   be given intravenously as prophylaxis.

7

Observation	Significance
Respiration (rate, rhythm and depth)	• Any depression in the rate or depth of respiration may indicate inadequate oxygen (see ans. 5).
Pulse and blood pressure	• There is an increase in the permeability of the capillaries after a burn. This results in a leakage of water, electrolytes and protein into the tissues, which continues for about 48 hours. Tachycardia and hypotension may indicate hypovolaemic shock as the heart pumps this smaller circulatory volume around the body.
Urine output	• Hypovolaemia means that there is a fall in renal circulation. Acute renal failure may ensue. • An hourly urine output of less than 30 ml per hour may indicate this. An hourly output also gives a guide to the amount of fluid to be infused.
Urine testing	• A high specific gravity may indicate inadequate fluid replacement. • Dark-coloured urine (dark red to black) indicates the presence of haemoglobin released from damaged red cells. Mannitol may be used to flush out the haemoglobin and to prevent obstruction of the renal tubules. • The presence of protein may indicate renal failure. • Glycosuria may indicate pseudo-diabetes caused by stress.

Intake	• An accurate record of fluid intake (together with output) will give a reliable indication of the patient's fluid balance. Hypovolaemia can be detected by a negative balance.
Temperature	• Damage to the outer layer of the skin makes the burn patient very susceptible to temperature changes. • Hyperpyrexia or hypothermia may be indications of severe infection.
Weight	• Initial weight loss represents catabolism. If it continues, inadequate nutrition may be the cause.

8   As a response to shock, fear and pain gastric dilatation and paralytic ileus occurs. There is also an increase in the secretion of gastric acid, and stress ulcers can form. A nasogastric tube will be passed initially to remove the stomach contents as aspiration of vomit is an additional risk. It also prevents abdominal distension during the period of paralytic ileus. Aspirate should be observed for fresh or altered blood which may indicate gastric ulceration.

When peristalsis has returned enteral feeding can commence, the volume of feed being gradually increased over 24 days. Parenteral feeding may be necessary.

The dietician will calculate Karen's requirements, which will be a high protein and high calorie intake. She will also require iron to overcome the anaemia caused by traumatic haemolysis of her red cells. Vitamin supplements, especially vitamin C, will aid healing.

9   As a burn heals the resultant scar shortens the wound, producing contracture. This can be minimized by:

• **Correct positioning** This ensures that Karen's body is in correct alignment. The neck should be extended with a roll, the arms extended in a supine position, and the axilla abducted to an angle of 90°. Her hands within their dressings will be immobilized and elevated. The metacarpal joint should be flexed with the interphalangeal joints straight and the thumb fully abducted.

• **Splinting** Badly burnt joints may be splinted to immobilize them in the optimum position.

- **Early immobility** Once the burns have begun to heal, joints can be put through a full range of movements. Unaffected joints should be fully exercised with the help of a physiotherapist and occupational therapist.

10   Karen should be taught how to accept the psychological responses following a severe burn. These responses should be explained to nurses caring for Karen, and to her husband. They are:
 1 fear of death
 2 denial
 3 withdrawal
 4 aggression

- Provide Karen and her husband with the opportunity to discuss her fears of death and/or disfigurement. An honest, open approach will help her to trust the staff.
- Re-establish independence as soon as possible. Respect Karen's individuality and self-worth. Allow her to become involved in planning her care whenever possible.
- Ensure that staff are warned not to let their facial expressions indicate the severity of her appearance. Relatives should also be warned of this.
- Explain the healing process to Karen and her husband, as follows:
 1 Scars will get redder and will then fade.
 2 Contractures can be stretched at a later stage.
 3 Skin grafts can be performed.
- Sensory deprivation is inevitable due to isolation techniques. It may be further aggravated by swelling of the face and eyelids, obscuring vision. The family should be encouraged to visit frequently to talk to Karen. Karen's allocated nurse should stay with her and orientate her to time and place. The radio may provide stimulus and orientation.
- In providing psychological care for Karen the nurse should be aware that she may also experience stress and frustration in trying to provide comfort and reassurance to a severely ill and disfigured patient.

  She should verbalize her stress to her peers, the ward sister, and her tutor. In some intensive care units psychological support is provided for the staff on a group basis.

2.2 Mr Bailey—a patient undergoing coronary artery bypass surgery

Mr Ray Bailey, aged 45 years, is a teacher of 'A' level maths in the upper school of his local comprehensive school. He is married with two teenage children. He smokes 10–15 cigarettes a day and is slightly overweight.

He went to see his doctor after he began to have frequent episodes of indigestion-like chest pain. The doctor thought that he might have an ulcer, but after listening to his description of the pain (not related to meals, always relieved by rest) he ordered an exercise ECG. This confirmed angina and Mr Bailey commenced propranolol and glyceryl trinitrate. Because of his age he was put on the waiting list for angiography.

He has now been admitted to the ward for coronary angiography.

1. What information will be obtained from Mr Bailey in order to plan his care?
2. How would you explain coronary angiography to your junior colleague?
3. Describe the role of the nurse before, during and after coronary angiography.

The coronary angiography revealed that Mr Bailey had over 50% stenosis of the left anterior descending artery, circumflex and right coronary artery. He was advised to have coronary artery bypass surgery.

4. How would the nurse describe these findings to Mr Bailey and how would she explain how surgery would help?

Mr Bailey is put on the waiting list for coronary artery bypass surgery and is readmitted 6 weeks later, 4 days before his surgery is planned.

5. What psychological preparation will Mr Bailey need before his surgery?

6   Describe Mr Bailey's specific physical preparation for surgery.

Mr Bailey's saphenous veins were used to bypass his narrowed
coronary arteries. The operation was uneventful and he was transferred
to the intensive care unit. On return to the unit he is ventilated and
has a central venous pressure line and infusion in the brachial vein to
replace the fluid lost and to administer drugs.

Two underwater seal drains are present and ECG electrodes connect
the patient to a cardiac monitor.

---

7   Explain the significance of the observations made on Mr
    Bailey in the immediate post-operative period.

8   How would you explain the measurement of central venous
    pressure to a junior colleague?

9   Patients are prone to infection after major cardiovascular
    surgery. Give reasons for this and outline the prevention of
    infection during Mr Bailey's post-operative care. How may
    infection be indicated?

10 Describe how the nurse may prevent Mr Bailey from developing confusion and/or depression post-operatively while
    in the intensive care unit.

2.2 Answers

1

> **Pain**
> - What activities invariably bring on an attack?
> - How does Mr Bailey manage his pain?
> - How can the nurse help him during an attack?
> - Does he have methods of preventing attacks?
>
> **Lack of understanding**
> - What does Mr Bailey know of his diagnosis?
> - What does he know about the reason for his admission?
>
> **Activities of daily living**
> - Does Mr Bailey's angina interfere with his activities of daily living
>   to the extent that he needs nursing intervention?
>
> **Anxiety**
> - Does Mr Bailey appear anxious or depressed about his condition,
>   admission or proposed investigation?
> - Does he want help or advice to reduce these worries?
>
> **Health education**
> - Is Mr Bailey aware of the hazards of smoking and obesity?
> - Does he want help or advice to reduce these hazards?

Using this information it is possible to identify Mr Bailey's problems and to produce a care plan which hopefully will overcome the problems and meet Mr Bailey's needs.

2 First ask your junior colleague to define coronary angiography. She should be able to recognize that this means an X-ray of the coronary arteries.

You can then proceed to explain that a catheter is introduced either into the brachial or the femoral artery. It is advanced via X-ray control into the ascending aorta. Dye is injected into the coronary arteries and a series of films is taken. These films demonstrate any blockage of the coronary arteries. The degree and position of such blockage will determine whether the damage is amenable to surgery.

The patient is not anaesthetized as normal cardiac function is necessary to accurately assess the coronary vessels, but a sedative is usually given to allay anxiety.

3 **Preparation for coronary angiography** Severe anxiety can cause vasoconstriction and prevent an accurate investigation, so it is essential to explain to Mr Bailey what the angiography entails. He will lie on a trolley under X-ray equipment in semi-darkness. A narrow tube will be passed through an artery in the crook of his left arm or in the groin. The tubing will be passed through this site up to the main artery supplying the heart. The doctors can watch the progress of the tubing via X-ray screens. Once the tubing is in place radiopaque dye will be injected into it. The dye will flow through the tubing and then into the arteries that supply the heart muscle. A series of X-rays will then be taken which will enable the doctors to detect the blockages that have caused his angina.

The procedure is lengthy but not painful. The most unpleasant part is the injection of the dye, which causes an uncomfortable burning sensation. A nurse will be at his side throughout the procedure and she will make every effort to reduce any discomfort by allowing him to talk about his concerns.

The following are also required for the preparation:
1 **consent** The patient should sign a consent form once the procedure has been explained to him.
2 **shaving** The left arm or groin should be shaved to avoid the introduction of infection.
3 **fasting** The patient should be starved for 4–6 hours prior to the procedure to reduce the risk of inhalation in the event of cardiac arrest.
4 **gown** In order to facilitate easy access to the arteries the patient should wear a theatre gown.

Care during the procedure The nurse should stay beside the patient's head throughout the procedure. She should try to reassure the patient by her calm and competent manner. She should also maintain a calm conversation to relax the patient and enable him to lie still during the investigation.

After-care This involves the following:
position
- The limb used for the initial incision should be kept straight to prevent turbulence of blood in the traumatized vessel and the formation of a thrombus. If the femoral artery has been used the patient will remain in bed for 12–18 hours.

observation
- Pulse in the affected limb should be observed quarter-hourly at first. A fast, weak pulse is indicative of haemorrhage. Bradycardia may result from poor perfusion to the

limb. If a blood clot obstructs the arterial flow, no pulse will be palpable.

- Perfusion can also be monitored by the observation of colour, temperature and sensation in the affected limb. A cold, pale, paraesthetic limb indicates poor perfusion, probably due to an embolus.
- Blood pressure should be recorded, initially quarter-hourly, as hypotension is a sign of haemorrhage.
- The wound should be observed quarter-hourly for bleeding as an arterial haemorrhage could be catastrophic. Swelling due to haematoma formation is another complication that should be watched for.
- Anaphylactic shock can occur as a result of an allergy to the radiopaque dye. Urticaria, flushing, nausea and vomiting, dyspnoea and hypotension may be indications of anaphylactic shock.

4 Draw a diagram of the heart to indicate the coronary arteries and show this to Mr Bailey (Fig. 6). The appropriate vessels can then be shaded in to demonstrate the blockages. Explain that stenosis means 'narrowing'.

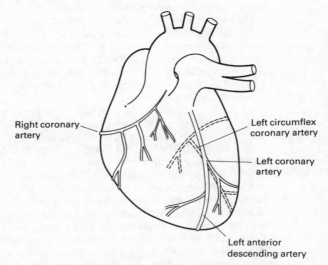

Fig. 6 The heart, showing the coronary arteries.

Then explain that surgery involves removing the saphenous vein from the leg. (This vein runs from the groin to the back of the knee. When this is removed blood simply uses other smaller veins and the blood supply to the leg is not affected.) The blocked parts of the coronary arteries can then be bypassed by lengths of the saphenous veins.

A heart–lung machine is used to circulate and oxygenate Mr Bailey's blood while his heart is being repaired.

Mr Bailey should be warned that although the surgery will overcome his angina, it is not a permanent cure. Stenosis can occur in the other coronary artery, so he should still take care to minimize the predisposing factors such as smoking and obesity.

5   Coronary artery surgery is well-known to the public nowadays, but Mr Bailey may have a distorted idea of what is involved.

The operation should be explained as above. The benefits and risks of the surgery should be given honestly.

Prior to surgery a nurse from the intensive care unit (ICU) should visit Mr Bailey and explain his immediate postoperative care and the equipment involved. Mr and Mrs Bailey may visit the ICU to see this equipment and to familiarize themselves with the unit. An explanation of assisted mechanical ventilation should be given.

Mr Bailey should be reassured that although he will be unable to speak while being ventilated, a nurse will be with him constantly and will be aware of any need for painkillers or sedation. He will probably only need ventilation for 6–12 hours after surgery, and will probably be asleep for much of this time.

Mr Bailey should be allowed time to express his fears and ask any questions. He may be reassured by meeting patients who have made uneventful recoveries from bypass surgery.

The hospital chaplain may also be helpful to Mr and Mrs Bailey in the pre- and post-operative period.

6   **Physiotherapy** Chest infection is a particular problem after cardiac surgery because of the sternal incision and immobility during ventilation. A visit from the physiotherapist enables the patient to practise deep breathing exercises and also to appreciate the need for these exercises.

Prevention of infection This involves the following:

- Shave his chest, arms and axilla to allow access to the operation site and cannulation sites.
- Shave his legs and groin for removal of the saphenous vein.
- Bath him and wash his hair with bactericidal soap.
- Take nasal and throat swabs and give antibiotics if necessary.

7

Observation	Significance
Ventilation	Poor colour (pallor or cyanosis) and/or shallow chest movement may indicate atelecasis or sputum retention.
Heart rate and rhythm	An apex rate of 90–120 beats/min is necessary to maintain cardiac output. A temporary pacemaker may be considered for a pulse below 80 beats/min. Tachycardia may be a sign of tamponade, heart failure, pain or anxiety. Arrhythmias may indicate electrolyte imbalance.
Blood pressure	Hypotension may be due to blood loss or heart failure. Hypertension may strain the suture lines and precipitate haemorrhage. It is commonly due to pain and anxiety.
Central venous pressure (CVP)	A low CVP indicates fluid loss. Blood may need to be transfused. A high CVP indicates overload of fluid, heart failure, or tamponade. Diuretics or further surgery may be required.
Temperature	Peripheral temperature should improve with cardiac output. Temperature is about 30°C on return from theatre but should return to normal within 6–8 hours. A falling temperature indicates shock due to fluid loss.
Level of consciousness	The patient should return to consciousness within an hour post-operatively. If the patient cannot respond to his name or move spontaneously after this time, a cerebrovascular accident may have occurred during the operation.

Wound drainage	Two underwater seal drains will be in situ. These should reduce wound drainage from 600 ml per hour to 50 ml per hour. It should also change to haemoserous fluid after about 6 hours post-operatively.
	Excessive fresh bleeding indicates haemorrhage.
	The drainage should also be observed for oscillation and free drainage, as a blocked tube could cause a mediastinal shift.
Blood transfusion	Sudden vasodilation and pulmonary oedema may indicate cardiac overload.
	A rash, pyrexia or rigor may be the result of a reaction to the tranfusion.
Fluid balance	An hourly urine output of less than 50 ml per hour may indicate incipient acute renal failure.
	After bypass surgery the output is usually high (400–500 ml per hour) for the first 4–6 hours post-operatively.

8 Ask your junior colleague if she knows what CVP measures. She should know that it is a measurement of the blood pressure within the right atrium.

You can explain that this measurement reflects blood volume, cardiac function and vascular tone.

CVP readings normally range from 5 to 15 cmH$_2$O. An elevated reading over 15 cmH$_2$O may be a sign of hypervolaemia, heart failure or vasoconstriction. A low reading (below 5 cm) may be due to hypovolaemia, angioneurotic oedema or vasodilation.

Other conditions also cause the CVP measurement to change. The junior nurse may be able to give some examples (pain, anxiety, respiratory rate). Therefore, one isolated CVP recording is of little value, but a series of correlated readings taken at 15 or 30 minute intervals provides a means of assessing the patient who is seriously ill.

Following the above explanation the junior nurse should accompany you to the bedside and observe the CVP measurement (see Fig. 7). She should be asked the possible significance of the result.

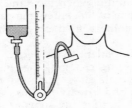

1 Check that the intravenous infusion is functioning.

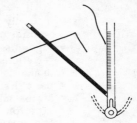

2 With the aid of a levelling stick ensure that the '0' level on the manometer is approximately level with the patient's right atrium.

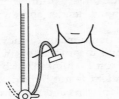

3 Turn the manometer stop-cock so that fluid enters the manometer.

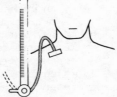

4 Turn the stop-cock to close off the intravenous infusion. Fluid from the manometer will enter the patient.

5 Take a central venous pressure reading at the highest point of oscillation when the fluid comes to rest. Having recorded the pressure return the stop-cock to the position shown in 1.

Fig. 7 Procedure for taking a reading of the central venous pressure (CVP).

9　Patients are particularly prone to infection after major cardiovascular surgery for the following reasons:
   - Body defences are reduced due to decreased peripheral circulation.
   - Infection can readily enter the circulation via intravenous cannulae and the lungs via the endotracheal tube or suction catheters.
   - Chest drainage tubes and the sternal wound offer organisms a chance to enter the thoracic cavity.

- A urinary catheter is present to facilitate assessment of renal function. Urinary catheters predispose to urinary tract infections.

The prevention of infection should be stressed to all personnel. Ways of prevention are:

- prophylatic antibiotics from pre-medication until 3–5 days post-operatively
- a strictly aseptic technique when handling the patient's wounds or any equipment that enters the patient's body.
- vigorous chest physiotherapy to prevent the stasis of secretions
- analgesia to allow the patient to cooperate
- use of humidifying tubing, changing the giving sets daily
- swabs taken on alternate days from the nose, throat, expectorated sputum and urinary meatus

The nurse should be alert for any signs of infection and should report them immediately. Infection may be indicated by:

- pyrexia, especially if accompanied by rigors
- purulent sputum and congested lungs
- an inflamed, discharging, tender and swollen wound or cannula site

10   A few patients who undergo major cardiovascular surgery experience confusion and disorientation in the early postoperative period. This can be minimized by:

- ensuring that the patient is not hypoxic
- giving adequate explanations and reassurance about procedure and equipment before surgery and before care is carried out
- eliminating unnecessary environmental stimuli such as noise or bright lights which interfere with sleep and rest
- anticipating the patient's needs
- providing adequate sedation and analgesia as prescribed

After most surgery many patients find tiredness such a problem that they become very depressed and even tearful about this constant lethargy. They may also be fearful of their condition.

Depressive feelings can be minimized by:

- preventing the feeling of isolation after transfer from the intensive care unit by remaining in view and providing a call-bell
- communicating with the patient about his progress
- providing rest periods during the day and planning care to ensure that these are adhered to
- advising visitors not to overtire the patient

- reassuring the patient that lethargy and tearfulness are not uncommon and that they will pass
- giving the patient time to talk about his fears and anxieties and to ask questions

2.3   Mr Simons—a young adult who has sustained a severe head injury

Mr Keith Simons, aged 28 years, has been brought into the accident and emergency ward following a car accident. He has sustained a head injury and is deeply unconscious on admission.

According to the ambulancemen he was conscious when they reached the scene of the accident but lost consciousness on the way to hospital.

Mrs Simons is with her husband. She is 8 months pregnant. Apart from being very shocked she is uninjured.

1   Describe the information required from the ambulancemen and Mrs Simons.
2   Describe how the nurse should assess Mr Simons' level of consciousness.
3   Explain the significance of the other observations to be made on Mr Simons.
4   How should Mrs Simons be cared for?

Mr Simons' condition rapidly deteriorates. His coma deepens and his left pupil becomes fixed and dilated. A CAT scan is carried out and reveals an extra-dural haematoma and gross cerebral oedema.

Intravenous dexamethasone 40 mg is ordered and an infusion of mannitol 20% 1–4 mg per kilogram body weight is prescribed to run over 30 minutes prior to surgery.

A burr hole is performed to evacuate the haematoma and a ventricular catheter is inserted to facilitate intracranial pressure monitoring.

Mr Simons is transferred to the intensive care unit and given assisted mechanical ventilation.

5   How should a CAT scan be explained to a junior colleague?
6   Explain why surgical intervention is of prime importance for Mr Simons.
7   Explain the advantage of using artificial ventilation in Mr Simons' care.
8   Using a problem-solving approach plan Mr Simons' care for the first 6 hours post-operatively.

9 Discuss how Mrs Simons can be reassured during Mr Simons' stay in the intensive care unit.

2.3   Answers

1   An accurate history will ascertain any change in the patient's condition before his arrival in hospital. It will also offer an assessment of the severity of the head injury.

Information required from the ambulancemen includes the following:

- When Mr Simons was conscious after the incident, was he confused or well orientated?
- How long was he conscious for? Was his loss of consciousness sudden or gradual?
- What movements did he make? Were they purposeful or were they suggestive of an epileptic fit?
- Have there been any vital signs since the incident? Have there been any significant changes in these signs?
- Are there any other injuries? How have these been treated?
- Is there any oozing of blood or clear fluid from the patient's nose and ears?
- What were his pupil size and reactions like immediately after the incident? Have these changed since then?

Mrs Simons is shocked and obviously not able to answer detailed questions at this stage. However, if possible the following are important facts to ascertain:

- Has Mr Simons being eating or drinking recently (danger of inhaling vomit)?
- Has he any chronic chest condition (that may predispose him to hypoxia)?
- Is he an epileptic or diabetic (conditions that may complicate assessment of his consciousness level)?

2   Proper assessment of the level of consciousness involves three phases:

1 eye opening
2 verbal response
3 motor response

Eye opening Note and record whether Mr Simons opens his eyes spontaneously, as a response to sound or a direct command, as a response to pain, or not at all. (Facial paralysis or trauma may prevent him from opening his eyes.)

Verbal response Note and record Mr Simons' ability to respond verbally. First see if he is alert or drowsy before speaking to him. If he is asleep is he difficult to rouse? Is he restless or irritable?

Then talk to him to assess his orientation to time and

space. Does he know who he is and where he is and the month and year? Or does he respond either inappropriately by groans or moans, or not at all?

Motor response Note and record Mr Simons' ability to move in response to commands. Does he respond to simple verbal orders? Or does he only move in response to painful stimuli? Is this movement purposeful to move away from the pain? Or is there no response at all?

Recordings should be specific. The record should include the stimulus used, how it was used and exactly how the patient responded. This type of report cannot be misinterpreted and can be easily compared with previous and future observations.

3

Observation	Significance
Respirations	Dyspnoea and/or cyanosis may indicate an obstructed airway or it may mean that the head injury has interfered with the respiratory centre in the brain stem.
Pulse	Bradycardia may be the result of a rise in intracranial pressure as a feature of brain stem compression.
Blood pressure	Hypertension may also be the result of brain stem compression. Hypotension may indicate blood loss.
Temperature	Hyperpyrexia can occur due to damage to the hypothalamus—the heat-regulating centre in the cerebrum. The hypothalamus can increase intracranial pressure as an increased body temperature increases cerebral metabolism. Permanent neurological damage may occur.
Pupil size and reaction to light	One dilated pupil fixed in its reaction to light may be due to an oculomotor nerve palsy from direct damage to the nerve. This abnormal observation would be present from the time of the head injury.

	If a pupil becomes gradually larger and more sluggish in its reaction to light this may be due to compression of the oculomotor nerve by an increase in intracranial pressure.
Motor function	Changes in limb power can be due to compression of a cerebral hemisphere due to cerebral oedema or haematoma formation.
	Fits may result from irritation to cerebral cells from intracerebral bleeding.

4 Mrs Simons should be allowed to lie down. She is shocked so a recumbent position will improve the cerebral blood flow and reduce the likelihood of fainting.

Someone should remain with her and explain that her husband is being looked after and that as soon as his condition has been assessed his doctor will speak to her. (Ensure that this occurs.) She will be able to see him as soon as is possible.

Meanwhile she should be encouraged to rest for the sake of her baby. She can be reassured that the baby is unharmed.

She can be asked if she would like a relative or friend to be with her.

5 Ask your junior colleague if she knows what the abbreviation CAT stands for (computed or computerized axial tomography).

You can proceed to explain that it involves the use of X-ray and computer equipment to distinguish between tissue densities in the brain.

The patient lies flat on a table with just his head inside a large, cap-like X-ray machine. During only a few minutes X-rays will be taken of the head from all angles and increasing depths. Readings are fed into a computer which distinguishes between brain, bone and fluid and produces a picture that indicates these various tissues.

CAT scans have the advantage of being a non-invasive investigation which can quickly reveal the size, position and content of the ventricles, and the degree and location of haematomas and cerebral oedema.

6 Cerebral oedema due to trauma and cerebral haematomas

causes a rise in pressure within the cranium. Intracranial pressure rises when any structure inside the skull expands because within the rigid skull there is no room for expansion.

Initially, some compensation occurs. Blood is pushed out of the intracranial veins into the systemic circulation. Then the cerebral tissue itself becomes compressed with a consequent loss of function.

If the pressure continues to rise the arteries become compressed, causing cerebral ischaemia, and the cerebral tissue is pushed out of the midline. This results in the compression of neurons and nerve tracts and, if left untreated, results in brain death.

Eventually, brain herniation occurs through the tentorial hiatus and downwards through the foramen magnum.

Thus, surgical intervention is of prime importance if the cause is known to be a haematoma in order to minimize brain damage and prevent herniation.

7   Head injuries cause inadequate ventilation in two ways. First, changes in the level of consciousness alter the ability to maintain a clear airway. Secondly, the trauma may have interfered with the respiratory centre in the brain stem. This results in reduced oxygen intake, cerebral anoxia and the retention of carbon dioxide which causes dilatation of the cerebral vessels. Cerebral anoxia and vasodilation both exacerbate raised intracranial pressure.

Artificial ventilation can provide a controlled inspired oxygen concentration to prevent the above from occurring.

8

Problem	Aim	Nursing care	Evaluation
Potential hypoxia (due to accidental disconnection from the ventilator, or mechanical failure)	To maintain artificial ventilation	• If alarm sounds look for disconnection or leak. • Leave slack in lines to allow for movement of patient. • Move patient carefully and slowly. • Monitor respiratory rate and colour. • Check ventilator settings 2–4 hourly.	No problems with ventilator and no dyspnoea or cyanosis observed

Potential airway obstruction	To ensure patency of the endotracheal tube	• Perform suction one hourly and when necessary. • Loosen secretions with humidification and normal saline instilled into the tube during suction (in conjunction with the physiotherapist).	Breathing not obstructed
Potential raised intracranial pressure (due to haemorrhage or oedema)	To be alert to any deterioration	• Make half-hourly neurological observations Report: 1 changes in level of consciousness 2 bradycardia and hypertension 3 hyperpyrexia 4 changes in pupil size and reaction to light 5 changes in motor response 6 epileptiform fits	No change in neurological observations
Potential corneal damage (due to loss of the corneal reflex)	To ensure that the corneas remain free from infection and trauma	• Keep eyes closed or apply moist eye pads. • Install normal saline eye drops as prescribed. • Swab eyes 2-hourly.	No signs of corneal infection or damage

Immobility	To ensure that hygiene needs are met	• Bed bath at least daily. • Ensure 2-hourly mouth care. • Ensure 4-hourly catheter care. • Position limbs to reduce contractures. • Change his position 2-hourly. • Observe pressure areas for redness and breakage of skin. • Perform passive limb exercises.	Skin, mouth and urethral meatus clean and healthy, and no signs of pressure sores or contractures.
Potential dehydration (due to the immobility of the patient, preventing him from taking fluids and nutrition)	To ensure patency of the infusion	• Check rate of infusion. • Immobilize cannula site. • Check cannula site for swelling, redness or leakage.	Intravenous infusion running to regimen
	To monitor the hydration status	• Measure intake and output.	Positive fluid balance observed
Lack of stimulus	To endeavour to stimulate a return to consciousness	• Explain all care. • Talk to patient while performing care. • Encourage visitors to talk to patient.	No response to communication
Inability to control elimination	To ensure normal elimination of urine	• Keep catheter patent.	Catheter draining well

9   Mrs Simons will be very frightened and anxious. She can be reassured by honest and frequent explanations of her husband's condition and treatment. She should be allowed to be with him whenever she wishes and she can be offered a bed in the hospital overnight.

It is important that she realizes that she must not become overtired and should be encouraged to have a good night's sleep and a daytime rest for her baby's sake. She should be reassured that she will be called whenever there is any change in her husband's condition.

She may also find it reassuring to be able to help in her husband's care. She may be able to help in caring for his hygiene. She can be told that just being with him, holding his hand, and talking to him may stimulate a return to consciousness as hearing is the first sense to return.

2.4   Mr Smith—a man who is to have a laryngectomy

Mr William Smith, aged 58 years, has been admitted to the ward for a laryngectomy. Two years ago he developed a cough and cold and lost his voice. Once his cold had cleared he was left with persistent hoarseness, in spite of the cough mixture he bought at the chemist's shop. He eventually went to his doctor who referred him to an ENT consultant. Indirect laryngoscopy revealed a tumour and he was given an early date to come into hospital for direct laryngoscopy and biopsy. The biopsy revealed a well-differentiated squamous cell carcinoma of the larynx, and a 6-week course of radiotherapy was organized.

Following the course of radiotherapy Mr Smith was seen monthly in the outpatient department. At his most recent visit he complained of dysphagia and weight loss. A further endoscopy and biopsy revealed a recurrence of his original tumour, and he is told of the need for surgery.

Mr Smith is a publican and is married with two married daughters. He smokes about 20 cigarettes a day.

1   What information will the nurse require from Mr Smith in order to plan his care?
2   Describe the information Mr Smith will require post-operatively.
3   While on night duty you observe Mr Smith smoking in bed. What should you do?
4   Describe Mr Smith's investigation and physical preparation prior to theatre.

Mr Smith's surgery consists of removal of his larynx, epiglottis, hyoid bone, thyroid and cricoid cartilages, and the first part of his trachea. The severed lower part of the trachea is brought up onto the skin surface as a permanent orifice. A laryngectomy tube is inserted into the orifice and suction drains are positioned on either side of this opening.

Following his operation Mr Smith is recovered in theatre and then transferred to the intensive care unit for the first 48 hours of his post-operative care.

5   Describe the maintenance of Mr Smith's airway in the immediate post-operative period.
6   How would you explain to your junior colleague the effect of Mr Smith's surgery on the anatomy and physiology of his respiratory tract?
7   Explain how Mr Smith's nutritional needs may be met during his post-operative care.
8   Describe how Mr Smith's communication needs may be met until he is ready for discharge.
9   Mr Smith makes an uncomplicated recovery and is ready for discharge in 3 weeks. What advice should he and his wife be given before he returns home?
10 Outline the education of the general public in relation to carcinoma of the larynx.

2.4 Answers

1

Social factors
- **Family** Is Mrs Smith alive and well? How dependent does Mr Smith seem to be on her? If the relationship is good, Mrs Smith may like to be included in carrying out care for her husband.
- **Personality** Does Mr Smith appear sociable, talkative or inhibited by his hospitalization? These traits may affect his reaction to surgery and the speed and motivation of his rehabilitation.
- **Occupation** Communication is a very important part of Mr Smith's job. Also, because oesophageal speech is difficult to hear in noisy environments, an artificial larynx may be the best method for him to adopt after surgery.
- **Education** How well does Mr Smith grasp details and information? His level of understanding and literacy will determine the level of your explanations before and after surgery.

Medical problems
- **Respiratory function** Does Mr Smith appear at all breathless or cyanosed? Chronic lung disease will interfere with his response to general anaesthetic as well as his ability to use oesophageal speech.
    Does he expectorate sputum? What colour is it? Chest physiotherapy may be planned to maximize respiratory function pre-operatively.
- **Smoking/drinking habits** Is Mr Smith aware of the dangers of smoking and drinking? Is further education needed or does he need help to give up these habits?
- **Oral hygiene** Does Mr Smith wear dentures? These need to be wellfitting to allow for oesophageal speech. Or does he have missing teeth or dental caries? Bad teeth will be treated pre-operatively and gaps in dentition will be noted as these may affect tongue movement in oesophageal speech.

Psychological factors
- **Reaction to condition** How does Mr Smith appear to react to his forthcoming surgery? Does he seem depressed or over-anxious? Help may be required pre-operatively.

---

2 **What the operation will entail** Diagrams (see Fig. 8) may be a useful way of easily teaching this aspect.
The effects of the surgery
- **Short term** he will return from theatre with a permanent hole in his neck which will prevent normal speech. At

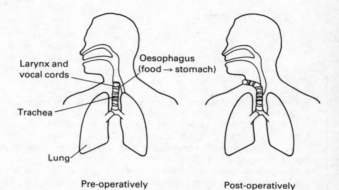

Larynx and
vocal cords

Oesophagus
(food → stomach)

Trachea

Lung

Pre-operatively   Post-operatively

Fig. 8   Diagram to show the results of a laryngectomy.

this stage communication will be via a bell, paper and pencil. Breathing and coughing will now occur via the opening in his neck. A lot of phlegm tends to be produced immediately after surgery which the nurse will remove by suction.

Two wound drains may be situated on either side of the opening. Also, a tube will be positioned in one nostril. This leads to the stomach and will be used for feeding until the internal wound has healed. An infusion or blood transfusion may also be present.

• **Long term** He will be taught alternative methods of communication by the speech therapist who he will meet pre-operatively. He may find that taste and smell are diminished, especially at first.

He should be reassured that normal life can be continued after surgery. If possible he should meet another patient who can describe his experiences and demonstrate oesophageal speech.

Post-operative equipment Mr and Mrs Smith should visit the intensive care unit and see some of the equipment that will be used post-operatively. Ideally, they may be able to meet the nurse who will be primarily looking after Mr Smith.

3   Talk to Mr Smith. Explain that smoking in bed is a fire risk that you cannot allow. Offer him the opportunity of sitting in the day room or stay with him while he smokes. Ask him why he is smoking; he probably cannot sleep, possibly due to his anxieties. Try to encourage him to talk about his worries.

After this conversation gently ask if Mr Smith is aware of the dangers of smoking. This may give him a further opportunity to talk. You may be able to offer help and reinforce the idea that laryngectomy offers a good cure rate and that smoking may hinder a good result.

4
- Urinalysis for glucose and protein to exclude diabetes and renal disease
- Chest X-ray to exclude pulmonary metastases
- Measurement of haemoglobin to ensure that a pre-operative transfusion is not necessary
- Grouping and cross-matching to ensure that blood is available for transfusion post-operatively
- Nasal and throat swabs to eliminate any pathogens. Any organisms other than normal flora will be treated with antibiotics.
- Sputum specimen to identify and treat any respiratory infection
- Electrolytes and urea to correct any imbalance due to poor nutrition because of dysphagia
- Deep breathing exercises to maximize the respiratory function will be carried out by the physiotherapist.
- Shave the beard area, neck and upper chest to prevent bacteria from infecting the area of surgery.
- Provide nil-by-mouth for 4–6 hours before surgery to prevent the inhalation of vomit under anaesthesia.
- Provide night sedation (e.g. temazepam) on the night before surgery to allay anxiety.
- Bath, provide a theatre gown, and remove any prosthesis prior to pre-medication to ensure cleanliness and safety in theatre.
- Give pre-medication (e.g. Omnopon 20 mg, hyoscine 0.4 mg) 1 hour before surgery to allay anxiety and to dry up secretions to facilitate nasal intubation of the tracheal tube.

5

Position	• Mr Smith should be sitting upright, supported by pillows, with a wall suction and oxygen by the bed.
Laryngectomy stoma	• Humidified oxgyen should be supplied via a tracheostomy mask.
	• Frequent suction should be

applied to remove mucus (approximately quarter-hourly) using an aseptic technique. Apply suction only on withdrawal of the catheter to avoid traumatizing the trachea. To prevent hypoxia apply suction for 5–10 seconds only at a time.

- Instil normal saline drops while suction is carried out to loosen secretion.

Monitor airway

- Observe Mr Smith for signs of dyspnoea or cyanosis.
- Also check his neck for any bleeding or swelling due to haematoma formation, either of which could obstruct the airway.

Prepare for potential complications

- In the event of an obstructed airway an extra tracheostomy tube of the correct size and a pair of tracheal dilators should always be at the bedside.

6   Ask your junior colleague to draw a diagram of the normal respiratory tract and explain the functions of each part.

You can then indicate how the anatomy of Mr Smith's respiratory tract has been altered by surgery. In relation to this explain how function has also altered, thus:

- The upper respiratory tract is no longer used, so filtering, warming and moistening of inspired air can no longer occur.
- The vocal cords have been removed, so normal speech is no longer possible. Crying, laughing and sighing are also affected.
- The loss of vocal cords also results in the inability to cough noisily.
- Air no longer involves the nasal passages or mouth and may lead to an impairment of taste and smell.
- Now that the nose is no longer involved in respiration, Mr Smith will not be able to sniff or blow his nose.

7   **Immediate post-operative period** Fluid intake is provided by an intravenous infusion.

24 hours after surgery Once nausea has abated, nasogastric tube feeds can commence. Initially these consist of 30 ml of water hourly, aspirating the stomach before the next feed to ensure that it is being absorbed. The amount can then be gradually increased and dilute feeds introduced. During the initial feeding Mr Smith should be observed carefully to ensure that a tracheo-oesophageal fistula has not developed. If this complication occurs, feed would be seen leaking out of the laryngectomy stoma. Mouth care should be given while he is unable to swallow to prevent a sore mouth, which may then delay normal eating.

4–7 days after surgery Once Mr Smith can swallow his own saliva, which usually occurs about 4 days after surgery, he can begin to take small amounts of fluid orally. As soon as he is able to tolerate this, the amount can gradually be increased. If fluid passes easily and no fistula has developed, the nasogastric tube can be removed and a soft diet commenced. Mr Smith's likes and dislikes should be taken into account to make this type of diet more appealing.

7–14 days after surgery Normal meals should be possible during the second post-operative week. Mr Smith should be warned not to overdistend his pharynx as this could result in fistula formation.

A high protein diet will help the healing process and enable Mr Smith to regain his lost weight.

8 **Immediate post-operative period** Mr Smith will be rendered completely speechless. The nurse should remain with him to reassure him. He should be encouraged to communicate either by writing on a pad or mouthing words or by a pointer board.

First post-operative week Mr Smith will still have to rely on the above methods of communication. The nurse should try to anticipate his needs and be patient so that he has time to express himself. The speech therapist will visit to demonstrate the injection inhalation and swallow methods for oesophageal speech. Mr Smith can practise injection and inhalation until he can swallow properly.

10–14 days post-operatively Once Mr Smith is eating normally and the pharynx and oesophagus are shown to function normally with no leakage, speech therapy can begin. Mr Smith will be taught oesophageal speech. An artificial larynx may be given to him at this stage but these are usually reserved for those patients who are too old or too ill to learn oesophageal speech.

The nurse should encourage Mr Smith to practise his oesophageal speech between his speech therapy sessions.

9 • He should avoid dry, smoky atmospheres.

- He should not use talcum powder after bathing because of the risk of inhalation.
- He should take care not to let water enter his trachea during bathing. He cannot go swimming.
- If he wishes to wear a scarf or cravat to camouflage his laryngostomy it should be made of smooth material.
- He should carry a card which states that in an emergency, resuscitation must be applied to his stoma.
- He should attend speech therapy and the outpatient department according to his appointment card.
- He should persevere with oesophageal speech exercises.
- He should avoid smoking.
- He should obtain further supplies of suction catheters, laryngectomy tapes, stoma bids and cleaning equipment for the laryngectomy tube from the chemist via his general practitioner's prescription.
- Laryngectomy clubs will provide Mr Smith and his wife with an opportunity to share problems.

10   The public should be aware of the following:
- If patients with cancer of the larynx are diagnosed and treated early, surgery is rarely necessary.
- Early symptoms are persistent hoarseness, or change of voice. The general practitioner should be consulted immediately.
- There is a clear relationship between heavy smoking and laryngeal cancer, probably due to the constant irritation of the larynx by smoke.
- There is some evidence to suggest that heavy drinking can also predispose to cancer of the larynx.

2.5 Miss Day—a young woman who has taken an overdose

Miss Tracy Day, aged 22 years, is a single girl living in digs in the centre of town. She is unemployed and has had difficulty in finding employment. She is a quiet, withdrawn girl who finds it difficult to make friends. She has also split up with her boyfriend.

She is brought into the accident and emergency department by ambulance, deeply unconscious having taken an overdose of aspirin. A gastric wash-out is performed in this department. She is then transferred to the intensive care department for haemodialysis as a blood test reveals a salicylate level of 900 mg.

1 Describe Tracy's immediate care when she is brought into the accident and emergency department.
2 Describe the precautions to be taken when Tracy has her gastric wash-out.
3 Explain to a junior colleague the purpose of haemodialysis for Tracy.
4 Explain the significance of the nursing observations carried out in relation to Tracy's haemodialysis.

Tracy begins to regain consciousness. Haemodialysis is discontinued and she is transferred to an acute medical ward. She remains quiet and withdrawn and unwilling to communicate.

5 How can the nurse maintain a safe environment for Tracy?
6 How will the nurse determine the depth of Tracy's depression?
7 Describe how the nurse might develop a trust relationship with Tracy.
8 Outline the reasons why Tracy may have attempted suicide.
9 How can the nurse help to develop Tracy's feeling of self-worth?
10 How can Tracy be helped to avoid further suicidal feelings after discharge?

2.5   Answers

1
- Tracy should be taken to the resuscitation area.
- The nurse should check that she has a clear airway.
- She should be transferred onto a trolley and placed in the recovery position. The head of the trolley should be tipped downwards to minimize the risk of asphyxia, and aspiration of the gastric contents.
- A history should be taken from ambulancemen together with their observations and any empty drug bottles.
- An assessment of Tracy's level of consciousness should be made and recorded.
- Tracy's vital signs should be taken and recorded, including pupil size and response to pain. Any dyspnoea and cyanosis may indicate the need for a guedel airway and oxygen administration.

2
- If the patient is, like Tracy, deeply unconscious, an anaesthetist should be present as intubation is required prior to the lavage.
- Oxygen and suction should be within easy reach and in working order.
- Emergency resuscitation equipment should be at hand in case of inhalation of vomit and respiratory arrest.
- The procedure should be carried out by a doctor or a trained nurse to reduce the likelihood of the stomach tube being passed into the lungs. The position of the tube should be checked prior to introducing fluid.
- Tracy should be positioned in the recovery position and the head of the trolley tipped downwards to minimize the dangers of inhalation of vomit.
- The amount of fluid entering and leaving the stomach should be measured carefully to ensure that all the fluid siphoned in has returned.
- The gastric contents should be examined for any obvious tablets and smell of alcohol to endeavour to confirm the substance taken.
- A specimen of gastric contents should be taken for laboratory analysis.

3   First, check that your junior colleague is aware of the principles of haemodialysis. Haemodialysis is a process designed to bring blood into contact with a semi-permeable membrane through which diffusion can take place. A solution (dialysate), in which the membrane is immersed, has a similar composition to plasma.

The patient's blood is removed from an artery and pumped through the artificial kidney. As the blood passes through the machine water, metabolic waste and toxins pass from the blood through the membrane into the dialysate. The dialysate is composed so that electrolytes will then pass into the blood as necessary. The cleansed blood is returned to the body via a vein.

In a temporary situation such as this, vascular access will be via a Schrivner shunt. (Tubing will be inserted by a surgeon to produce an artificial communication between an artery and a vein or by direct cannulation.)

Because it is an acid, aspirin (salicylic acid) produces an excess of acid in the bloodstream, causing a metabolic acidosis. This can be overcome by the kidneys excreting more hydrogen ions to compensate for the excess acid in the extracellular fluid.

However, Tracy has an exceptionally high salicylate level which could be very toxic to the brain if it is not reduced quickly. Forced alkaline diuresis is one form of treatment—an infusion of alkalines at a high rate is given to encourage a rapid diuresis to quickly excrete the excess acid.

Haemodialysis, where available, is an even more efficient method of producing a rapid excretion of the acid via the dialysis machine.

4

Observation	Significance
Weight before and after dialysis	This determines the degree of fluid overload (i.e. the degree of overhydration) if the patient is markedly overweight after dialysis. A loss of weight may indicate dehydration.
Blood pressure	This also monitors the state of the patient's hydration. Hypotension may be the result of hypovolaemia and dehydration.
Temperature	A pyrexia may be caused by infection from sterile pathogens being washed into the patient.

Respiratory rate	Hyperventilation occurs as a result of metabolic acidosis. As dialysis progresses the respiratory rate should decrease as the blood pH returns to 7.4.
Level of consciousness	Extreme acidosis results in coma. As the dialysis progresses, Tracy's level of consciousness should rise.
Patency of shunt	This should be checked after dialysis. If blood cannot be seen to flow through the shunt, or if it feels cold to the touch, clotting has occurred.

5
- Provide supervision for Tracy when she is out of bed.
- Do not allow Tracy out of the ward area unless she is accompanied by a member of staff.
- Ensure that Tracy has nothing that she could use to harm herself (e.g belt, knife). Restrict or monitor the use of cigarettes, matches or lighter.
- Be alert to potentially dangerous objects such as glass vases or bottles, which should not be left in Tracy's possession.
- Tracy's bed should be positioned near the nurses' station but also away from exit doors.
- Tracy should be accompanied when she is attending to hygienic needs such as bathing and cutting nails.
- Observe Tracy carefully when giving her any medication to ensure that she actually swallows them and does not save them up.
- Do not leave medications, cleaning fluids, etc., unattended when unlocked. Ensure that keys are kept with the nurse-in-charge.

6   Tracy should be observed for the following signs of depression:
- sleep disturbances (early wakening, insomnia)
- disturbance of appetite (anorexia, excessive eating, weight loss or gain)
- problems with elimination (constipation)
- neglect of hygiene needs
- decreased motor activity or restlessness, and agitation
- decreased communication
- expression of suicidal ideas or behaviour (suicidal ges-

tures, self-destructive tendencies, talk about suicide plans)
- expressions of guilt feelings or unworthiness

7   One primary nurse should be allocated to care for Tracy. This nurse should:
- preferably have had previous experience with overdose patients
- be consistent and honest with Tracy
- accept Tracy as a person
- give positive feedback for acceptable or positive behaviour
- offer alternatives to negative or unacceptable behaviour
- help Tracy to identify the reasons for her suicide attempt
- provide support and companionship
- encourage Tracy to talk about her feelings
- be alert to detect Tracy's non-verbal signals
- convey an interest and a caring attitude by remaining with Tracy when she does not want to talk

8   Suicide is one of the ten commonest causes of death and its incidence is increasing among people aged 15–24 years.

Some of the commonest reaons for attempting suicide, which may be reasons for Tracy deciding to take an overdose, are:
- living away from one's family with no-one to share your problems.
- loss of employment, resulting in a loss of purposeful activity. The resultant loss of income may make alternative leisure activities unavailable.
- inability to gain employment, causing feelings of unworthiness and failure with loss of confidence (which may be relieved by a permanent job).
- break-up of a stable relationship which may add to the above feelings
- inability to make and maintain friendships, which may make one feel insecure and unwanted as well as aggravating one's feelings of low self-esteem and loneliness

9
- Accept Tracy as a person. Let her realize that you consider her a worthwhile person.
- Involve Tracy in planning her own care.
- Help her to identify positive aspects about herself and her life.
- Encourage her to express her feelings and accept these expressions without judgement.
- Encourage her to be involved in ward activities and give her opportunities to succeed in these.

- Allow her to make her own decisions but provide a supportive structure to the day.

10   Before discharge the nurse should carry out the following:

- Discuss Tracy's future plans with her. Explore possible employment alternatives.
- Decide how Tracy will cope with situations that have precipitated suicidal feelings in the past. She should be able to recognize the onset of such feelings and ideally have someone she can contact to help her alleviate such emotions.
- Talk about any changes that can be made in Tracy's lifestyle to decrease the likelihood of suicidal feelings.
- Give her a name and telephone number to contact in case of emergency (e.g. self-help groups, Samaritans).
- Provide some means of continued support (community psychiatric nurse or outpatient follow-up).
- Help Tracy to discover self-help groups in the community to avoid feelings of isolation or loneliness.

3 Care of the Patient with Problems of Body Image

3.1   Mrs Carpenter—a woman having an abdominoperineal resection

Mrs Joyce Carpenter, aged 62 years, was admitted to the ward a week ago for investigation of a possible carcinoma of the colon. She had been suffering from alternating bouts of diarrhoea and constipation with blood in the stools for some time, but had only recently sought help from her doctor.

A sigmoidoscopy and biopsy has confirmed carcinoma of the sigmoid colon and rectum, and abdominoperineal resection is to be performed in 2 days time.

Mrs Carpenter is happily married and has two children, both of whom are married. Mr Carpenter is due to retire soon and they have been busy planning a long-awaited extended visit to her sister who lives in Canada.

1   What effect may the forthcoming operation have on Mrs Carpenter's perception of her body image?
2   Outline a teaching plan that will help Mrs Carpenter to come to terms with her altered body image.
3   How would you explain the forthcoming operation to the junior nurse assigned to work with you?

Mrs Carpenter's surgery goes ahead as planned. She returns to the ward with an intravenous infusion and nasogastric tube in situ. She has a Foley urinary drainage catheter and wound drains to both the perineal and abdominal wounds.

4   Using a problem-solving approach describe the nursing care Mrs Carpenter will require in relation to her stoma for the first 48 hours following surgery.
5   What actions can the nurse take to promote Mrs Carpenter's comfort in the first few days post-operatively?

As Mrs Carpenter has an end-sigmoid colostomy, it will be possible for her to develop some bowel control. This can be achieved by altering her diet to suit her own individual needs and by introducing routine irrigations of her stoma.

6 What dietary advice should Mrs Carpenter be given that will help her to control her bowel movements?
7 Describe the principles of routine stoma irrigation.

Mrs Carpenter recovers very well following her surgery and hopes to be discharged after 2 weeks.

8 What advice can Mr and Mrs Carpenter be given with regard to:
(a) their proposed visit to Canada?
(b) their sex life?
(c) her convalescent period?

3.1 Answers

1   Mrs Carpenter may well see herself as 'unclean' and 'dirty' and therefore socially unacceptable. A fear of smell and wind will add to her shame.

    She may see herself as unacceptable to others and may not want other people to look at her, even though the stoma cannot be seen.

    She will probably see herself as unattractive and abnormal. She will consider that she is sexually unattractive and may not want her husband to look at her.

    She may feel that her children will see her differently. She may feel that she is no longer 'whole' and therefore that she is no longer the same mother figure.

2   Teaching should begin pre-operatively. There should be one nurse allocated to Mrs Carpenter who is responsible for teaching. The nurse must be able to cope with her own feelings towards stomas and must not show any repulsion or disgust. The plan should be developed with Mrs Carpenter and a reflective technique should be used to assist her in discussing her feelings and fears. The nurse should assess Mrs Carpenter's pre-operative approach to her body image in order to highlight any areas that may affect her acceptance of her altered body image.

Pre-operative teaching

- With the use of diagrams, teach Mrs Carpenter about her internal organs. Clear up any misconceptions she may have.
- Find out what she understands about the operation. Using diagrams again, show her how her internal organs will have altered post-operatively.
- Use a reflective technique to encourage her to talk about her problems.
- Introduce her to the stoma nurse who may possibly arrange for Mrs Carpenter to meet somebody who has had the operation.
- Give Mrs Carpenter appropriate books to read.
- Include general pre-operative teaching as for any other surgery.
- Assess Mrs Carpenter's level of understanding/learning by asking questions.

Post-operative teaching

- Begin as soon as possible. Teaching sessions should always be short and may need to be repeated.

- Mrs Carpenter's basic physiological needs must be met before she can be receptive to learning anything.
- First explain stoma care as you perform it, giving reasons for each step.
- Encourage Mrs Carpenter to look at the stoma while you are dressing it.
- Gradually involve Mrs Carpenter in day-to-day care—first, emptying her appliance, then caring for her skin, and finally applying her appliance herself.
- Encourage Mrs Carpenter and give positive feedback.
- Introduce her to the various possible appliances.
- Assess learning by watching Mrs Carpenter carry out care.
- Allow her to practise.
- Give time for her to ask questions and advice about care after discharge.
- Document all that is taught.
- Include Mr Carpenter in all teaching.

3 Find out what she has already been told or what she knows about the relevant anatomy and physiology and the proposed surgery.

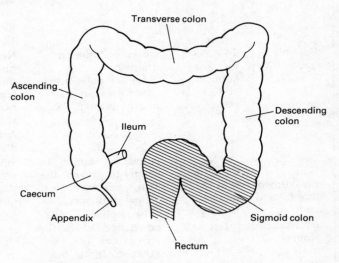

Fig. 9 The large bowel.

Draw a diagram of the large bowel (Fig. 9); the shaded area of the figure indicates the site of Mrs Carpenter's carcinoma.

An abdoperineal resection involves the removal of the entire anus, rectum and sigmoid colon. This will leave Mrs Carpenter with a permanent end-sigmoid colostomy.

The operation involves two surgeons. One surgeon works via an abdominal incision to resect the sigmoid colon and form the colostomy; the other surgeon works via the perineum to free the anus and rectum. Mrs Carpenter will therefore have two major wounds.

4

Problem	Goal	Nursing action	Evaluation
Possible circulatory failure to the stoma	To recognize the signs as soon as possible	Check stoma during first 24 hours for: • colour • drainage • size of stoma	Stoma bright red; only small serous drainage; no change in size of stoma.
Possible haemorrhage	To detect its occurrence as soon as possible	Observe stoma and drainage. Monitor pulse and blood pressure half-hourly until stable.	No bleeding; pulse and blood pressure within normal limits.
Possible skin breakdown due to acid and enzymes in stoma drainage, and irritation from bag	For Mrs Carpenter's skin to remain healthy and intact	Appliance should fit snugly to prevent the skin being exposed to stomal drainage. The appliance must be changed at the first sign of any leakage. When changing the bag, cleanse the skin with warm water and dry well. Apply a protective barrier to the skin before applying bag, e.g. Stomahesive	Skin around stoma is pink, healthy and shows no signs of irritation.

5
- Administer post-operative analgesia as prescribed at regular intervals to keep Mrs Carpenter free of pain.
- Help to position Mrs Carpenter in the most comfortable position, which is likely to be on either side because of the perineal wound.
- Change her position at least every 2 hours.
- Ensure that she is not lying on the wound drains or on the urinary drainage catheter.
- Make use of sheepskins and bedcradles.
- Fasten the nasogastric tube so that it is not pulling (using hypo-allergenic tape).
- Use pillows to support her arm with the intravenous infusion and to support her back and limbs.
- Administer mouth care while her fluids and diet are restricted.
- Give Mrs Carpenter a wash. Change her bedding post-operatively and then at least twice daily or as required.
- Plan care so as to perform activities when Mrs Carpenter has had her analgesia, and to allow her to rest.

6 There is no need for Mrs Carpenter to change her diet drastically but she should experiment and find those foods that she tolerates well. She should eat regular meals and avoid nibbling in between meals. She should try to avoid those foods that produce loose stools or flatus. She may be given a diet sheet which indicates these types of foods. For example she should avoid or take carefully:
- spicy foods
- onions
- some root vegetables/green vegetables
- pulses
- some drinks, e.g. beer, lager, fizzy drinks
- sugar

Some foods when eaten together cause flatus and odour, so she will have to experiment with these.

All foods must be chewed adequately to avoid undue flatus and odour.

She must take sufficient fibre to produce a firm stool. If the stool needs firming up then she may find 'bulkers' useful. These are non-drugs which form bulk and help to make the stool firmer. These may be useful for Mrs Carpenter until she learns to control her stools by diet alone.

The dietician should give Mrs Carpenter the chance to ask questions. Mr Carpenter should also be involved as he may well be preparing her meals initially.

7 Stoma irrigation involves instilling 500–2500 millilitres of

water (depending upon toleration) into the stoma. The build-up of pressure against the walls of the colon stimulates muscular contractions which then evacuate the bowel. If done routinely, at the same time every day, irrigation will empty the bowel and prevent stoma actions between irrigations.

8 (a) There is no reason at all why they should not go on their long-awaited holiday, though it may have to be delayed a little until Mrs Carpenter's perineal wound has healed and she is properly recovered from the operation. A holiday will do her good and will help to boost her confidence. As she will be staying with her sister it is important that she explains the nature of her operation so that her sister knows what to expect. Travelling should not pose a problem; she will be able to manage the stoma sufficiently well by that time to cope with air travel.

She will be able to obtain supplies in Canada and should take a letter from her doctor and then approach a doctor or hospital in her sister's town.

The Colostomy Association will be able to send her information about travelling.

(b) Explain that they can continue with their sex life as before, and that there is no reason why they should abstain. Mrs Carpenter may find her vagina a little tight at first but with relaxation this problem should be dispelled. In the initial post-operative period, when intercourse will be too painful due to the perineal wound, the couple can demonstrate their love and caring by other means.

If Mrs Carpenter is worried that her stoma may function during intercourse she can cover it with a stoma cap or dressing. It may help for them to talk to other couples in the same position. Sexual counselling can be obtained from an organization known as SPOD (Sexual and Personal Relationships of the Disabled).

(c) As her perineal wound may take some time to heal she should continue with normal saline baths at home. A district nurse will attend to inspect the wound and apply dressings if necessary.

She should avoid all heavy work and lifting that may predispose to prolapse of the stoma. She should have plenty of rest but should also begin to get some fresh air and begin short walks to exercise her legs. Help may be obtained in the form of a home help who will visit daily.

Mrs Carpenter should be looking after herself and the stoma as soon as possible after arriving home. Mr Carpenter should not do everything for his wife as this will prevent her from adapting her life.

3.2 Suzannah Michael—an adolescent with anorexia nervosa

Suzannah Michael, aged 17 years, has been admitted to the ward with severe anorexia nervosa.

Suzannah is the eldest daughter of an apparently happy family. She has one sister and one brother, both of whom are doing very well at school.

Suzannah is a boarder at a large ballet school. On a recent visit home her mother noticed that she appeared to have lost a lot of weight. When questioned about this, Suzannah denied being ill.

Eventually Suzannah was referred to the school doctor by her teacher who found her vomiting after meals on several occasions. On examination Suzannah was found to weigh only 35 kg. She had swollen ankles, sunken eyes, a subnormal body temperature and a pale, sallow complexion. Her last period had been over 6 months ago.

1 How can the nurse establish an effective relationship with Suzannah after admission?
2 Explain why Suzannah denied her weight loss even though it was quite obvious to others.
3 Briefly describe the factors that may have led to Suzannah's anorexia.
4 With reference to altered physiology how should Suzannah's symptoms be explained to a junior nurse?

As Suzannah's condition is critical the first aim of management must be to save her life. An intravenous infusion is commenced and strict bed rest implemented. As her general condition improves, so the psychiatrist becomes more involved in her care. The main aims of management now are to:
(a) help Suzannah to increase her weight to within 90% of her ideal weight
(b) establish normal eating behaviour
To achieve the first of these aims a system of rewards and privileges is introduced.

5 Explain the principles of this type of behaviour modification therapy.

6 What type of behaviour must the nurse be alert for while caring for Suzannah?
7 How should Suzannah's family be involved in her care and be helped to accept the apparently harsh therapy?

Suzannah is going to be in hospital for some time until she is finally discharged home. Throughout that time psychotherapy and family therapy will continue.

8 What are the possible long-term consequences of Suzannah's anorexia?

3.2   Answers

1
   - One nurse should be assigned to Suzannah as a key worker.
   - The nurse should have come to terms with her own attitude towards anorexia nervosa and have a positive body image.
   - She should spend time explaining the treatment regimen.
   - She should encourage Suzannah to talk about her fears and feelings.
   - She should talk about positive and healthy topics, e.g. hobbies, dancing school.
   - She must be honest, open, patient, dependable and consistent.
   - She must be firm yet supportive and understanding.
   - It is essential that she is non-judgemental.
   - All staff must be aware of the treatment regimen and should avoid manipulation by Suzannah.
   - Suzannah's key worker should be the one who is involved in any discussion concerning her therapy.

2   Suzannah will have a strong fear of gaining weight. Although she is severely emaciated she will see herself as fat and overweight, even when she looks in a mirror. This distorted body image makes it difficult for her to have any insight into her problems. She will go to great lengths to avoid putting on weight, as any weight gain will make her feel guilty and disgusted. She may be ashamed of her attitudes towards eating and of her behaviour. It is for these reasons that Suzannah will deny that she is ill and will have a general disregard for her basic nutritional needs.

3   There are many factors that may predispose to a young person developing anorexia nervosa. These include the following:
   - Current cultural pressures. Today great importance is placed on being slim. Advertisements show slim young women wearing up-to-date fashions.
   - The individual has a desire for personal autonomy and physical attractiveness. Being in control of your eating pattern and weight means meeting this desire.
   - Suzannah may have found it difficult to cope with the stress of being separated from her home and parents.
   - Ballet dancers tend to be below the average weight and she may be worried about putting on too much weight in case she has to leave the school.

- There may have been problems within the family, and possibly marital tensions. Her mother may have been over-protective, resulting in a sense of ineffectiveness in Suzannah.
- An inability or fear of coping with the demands of sexual maturity. Keeping thin is a way of avoiding menstruation and normal growth.
- Individuals are often very self-critical and obsessed with themselves.

4

Symptom	Related physiology
Amenorrhoea	Menstruation is controlled by hormones which, in turn, are controlled by the hypothalamus. The hypothalamus secretes gonadotrophic-releasing hormone which, in the years before puberty, is released in surges throughout the day. When the child's body reaches a critical weight she menstruates for the first time. If the body weight falls below that critical weight, as in anorexia nervosa, the hypothalamus fails to release the releasing hormones in sufficient amounts to bring about menstruation.
Swollen ankles	An insufficient intake of protein causes the osmotic pressure to be reduced, causing excess tissue fluid formation—oedema. The oedema will be dependent, i.e. in the ankles.
Subnormal body temperature	In a starved state the body tries to preserve energy by reducing the basal metabolic rate. This results in a lowered temperature and also a low blood pressure and pulse rate.
Sunken eyes and a pale, sallow complexion	These are signs of dehydration, which may be due to bone marrow suppression and anaemia.

5 Behaviour modification works on trying to change/modify behaviour by giving rewards or privileges when Suzannah reaches her target weight or shows positive eating behav-

iours. Although this method has its drawbacks it is still used by many units.

Usually during the initial period the individual is confined to bed. As Suzannah's weight increases, so she will be given rewards or privileges. For example:

- she may be allowed out of bed to use the lavatory, to have a bath, to use the telephone, or to dress and be up all day.
- she may be allowed to spend a weekend at home, go for a walk, or watch the television.

At first she will not be allowed any visitors. Visiting is a privilege that she must win by gaining her target weight.

6   The nurse must be constantly observant for any deceptive behaviour from Suzannah which might involve:

- trying to give false weight readings by stuffing objects into shoes or pockets, by drinking a lot of water from any source before being weighed, or by not passing urine for many hours
- hiding food under the pillow or blankets, then later disposing of it out of the window, with the rubbish, or down the lavatory
- inducing vomiting after having eaten, especially if left alone after a meal. She may vomit into toilets, washbasins, tissues or even clothing
- trying to obtain laxatives from other patients or attempting to conceal them on admission
- binging to increase weight, followed by self-induced vomiting
- bargaining with the nurses

7   Family therapy is extremely important as the problem often has its roots in family relationships. There should be sufficient family sessions to give all members the chance to solve problems that may have been highlighted. The parents should be clear about the treatment, especially during the first week or so when visiting is not allowed. They must be prepared to give the hospital staff support. They should feel happy with the treatment, as should Suzannah, and if they find it too harsh they should be allowed to seek alternative treatment. They should be kept informed of the progress Suzannah is making at all times. The reasons for separating Suzannah from her family should be explained. Suzannah is on neutral ground away from all the demands being made on her, and will be able to meet and talk to other people and form opinions uninfluenced by others.

The reasons for Suzannah's behaviour should be

explained to her parents and they should be told that once she regains weight her general attitude will improve. Once Suzannah has gained her target weight the family will be involved in therapy sessions during which time everybody is given a chance to talk about problems. When Suzannah is ready for discharge, home visits may be gradually introduced to give the family a chance to accept Suzannah back amongst them.

8
- Eighty per cent of individuals continue to have psychological problems, i.e. depressive/obsessional characteristics.
- Some individuals go on to develop bulimia (insatiable appetite), which holds a poor prognosis.
- Suzannah may continue to have an abnormal attitude to food and eating.
- Menstruation may take some time to return and may be irregular at first.
- There may be long-term renal and bowel complications due to self-induced vomiting and the possible use of laxatives.
- Suzannah will probably have excessive dental caries due to the acidity of the vomitus.
- Development may be stunted due to starvation during growth spurts. She may also have mild vitamin deficiencies.

3.3   Mrs Fitzgerald—a woman having a mastectomy

Mrs Mary Fitzgerald, aged 38 years, has been admitted to the ward for a right modified radical mastectomy. Mr Fitzgerald is a director of a large company and the couple have two children aged 6 and 4 years.

Mrs Fitzgerald gave up her job when her first child was born. She leads an active life, swimming at least three times a week and playing squash with her husband and friends at the week-end.

Mr Fitzgerald's mother is coming to stay to look after the children while her daughter-in-law is in hospital. The diagnosis of cancer of the breast was made three days before admission, so Mrs Fitzgerald has had a little time to think about the operation.

1   Discuss the importance of the nurse's initial nursing assessment of Mrs Fitzgerald.
2   How can the nurse help to prepare Mrs Fitzgerald for the forthcoming change to her body image?
3   With reference to normal and altered physiology what would you tell the junior nurse about Mrs Fitzgerald's operation?

Mrs Fitzgerald returns from theatre with a wound drain and an intravenous infusion in situ. She recovers well and is taking fluids and a light diet the day after surgery. The infusion is discontinued and on the third post-operative day the wound drain is removed.

One of the main nursing goals post-operatively is for Mrs Fitzgerald to be able to move her arm fully.

4   Outline a plan of exercises that will help Mrs Fitzgerald to regain full use of the affected side and arm.
5   How might Mrs Fitzgerald's body image be altered by the surgery and how can she be helped to adjust to her new image?
6   How can the nurse assess Mrs Fitzgerald's degree of acceptance of her altered body image?

Mr Fitzgerald visits regularly and is very anxious to be as supportive as he can.

7   What can the nurse do to help Mr Fitzgerald assist in his wife's rehabilitation?

On one of his visits Mr Fitzgerald asks how he and his wife should cope with the children's questions about their mother's hospitalization. The family have always been very open and the children are used to seeing both their parents without any clothes on.

8   What might be your response to the above question?

Mrs Fitzgerald is discharged 10 days post-operatively and an appointment is made for her with the radiotherapist, who recommends a 6-week course of radiotherapy to her right axilla. This course of treatment commences 5 weeks after the initial surgery.

9   What advice can the nurse give Mrs Fitzgerald to help her cope with some of the possible problems that might arise as a result of radiotherapy?
10 State briefly how Mrs Fitzgerald can be helped to come to terms with her altered body image during the first few months following successful therapy.

3.3 Answers

1 The initial nursing assessment is extremely important as it:
   - enables the nurse to find out exactly what Mrs Fitzgerald understands about the forthcoming surgery and its effects
   - allows the nurse to observe her closely for her reactions, noting whether she is openly anxious, hiding her fears, or feeling hopeless or resentful
   - gives the nurse a chance to clarify any misconceptions
   - should encourage Mrs Fitzgerald to ask questions and talk about the situation
   - enables the nurse to begin to build up a trusting relationship with Mrs Fitzgerald
   - should highlight any particular social problems, e.g. care of the children, that may need easing
   - allows the nurse to find out Mrs Fitzgerald's normal daily routine so that care can be individualized
   - enables the nurse to observe Mrs Fitzgerald's general state of health

2 - Explain the operation and what it entails. Make use of diagrams and/or pictures.
   - Explain what the wound will look like after surgery to clarify any misconceptions; if appropriate show her a picture.
   - The mastectomy nurse should meet Mrs Fitzgerald once or twice before surgery. She can talk to her about prosthesis and how she will be able to resume her normal lifestyle.
   - If appropriate Mrs Fitzgerald can be introduced to another woman who has had a mastectomy, preferably someone who has come to terms with the operation.
   - Mr Fitzgerald should be involved in all discussions.

3 Explain the position of the lymphatic glands and their function in relation to the female breast.

   Cancer cells spread from the original tumour via the lymphatic system to the lymphatic glands.

   A modified radical mastectomy removes all breast tissue and also the pectoralis minor muscle and axillary lymph nodes. The pectoralis major muscle is retained (see Fig. 10).

4 Exercises are usually begun by the fourth post-operative day. Mrs Fitzgerald must have adequate analgesia to ensure that exercises are pain free.

   During the first few post-operative days, encourage Mrs Fitzgerald to flex and extend her fingers, hand and forearm several times a day.

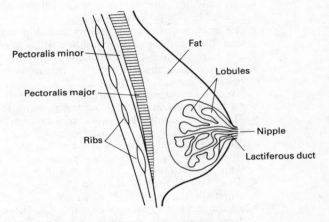

Fig. 10 Structure of the normal breast.

Begin exercises slowly and increase them according to Mrs Fitzgerald's tolerance. Encourage her to participate in the performance of self-care activities including: washing her face, cleaning her teeth and brushing her hair. All of these exercises encourage use of the arm.

A formalized exercise plan should include:

- **Wall-climbing exercises** Facing the wall, with palms of the hands against the wall, gradually move hands up the wall until they are fully extended.
- **Rope exercise** Circling a rope encourages circumduction of the arm.
- **Rope-pulling exercises** Throw a rope over a door or shower rail. Taking an end in each hand, pull the rope in a see-saw motion.

The physiotherapist will plan the formal exercises but the nurse must encourage Mrs Fitzgerald to perform these and other exercises. A written plan of exercises should be given to Mrs Fitzgerald when she goes home.

5   • Mrs Fitzgerald may feel that her womanhood has been lost.
- She may think that her identity as a woman has been disturbed.
- She might think that she no longer looks attractive and that other people will look at her in a different light, being able to tell that she has had a mastectomy.

- She may feel that her husband will no longer want to look at her or make love to her.
- She may worry about finding suitable clothes, feeling that those she must wear are less attractive.
- She may see herself as abnormal.
- Her role as a mother may be threatened as she fears rejection by her children.

Mrs Fitzgerald needs continued support from her husband and family and also from the nursing staff.

- The nurse should be aware of her own feelings and reactions to her altered body image.
- The nurses should not show any repulsion or distaste when changing her dressing; patients look for the reactions of others.
- Give Mrs Fitzgerald time to discuss her feelings; the nurse should listen with empathy.
- Encourage her to wear make-up, visit the hospital hairdresser and wear pretty nightclothes. These will help to emphasize her femininity.
- Encourage Mrs Fitzgerald to look at the wound once the drains are removed. Accept that she may need time to feel ready for this.
- Fit her with a temporary prosthesis as soon as possible.
- Encourage the family to visit as often as possible.
- If it has not been done pre-operatively, introduce Mrs Fitzgerald to another mastectomy patient.
- The mastectomy nurse will talk to her about her future care.
- Mrs Fitzgerald should be given the Mastectomy Association address.

6   Factors that indicate that she is beginning to cope include:
- a willingness to look at the wound and touch the changed area
- a willingness to let others look at the area
- an indication of wanting to participate in the care of the area
- a willingness to take over care of the area

Factors that may indicate a difficulty in coping include:
- not wanting to look at the wound
- being afraid to touch the area
- asking nothing about the care of the area
- being unwilling to talk about the operation

7
- Involve Mr Fitzgerald in all discussions from the beginning.
- Explain to him that his wife may exhibit depression or

swings of mood; knowing this is normal will help him to act appropriately.

- Involve him in teaching his wife her exercises so that he knows what she should be doing at home.
- Encourage him to be positive and to not show distaste of his wife.
- If possible encourage him to look at the wound during a dressing before discharge. This may help him to overcome the initial shock in hospital, where he will be able to talk about his reactions.
- Explain how he can give practical help at home (e.g. with heavy lifting) without allowing his wife to become an invalid.
- He should encourage her to socialize and he should be able to recognize when she has taken pains with her appearance.

8 They should explain Mrs Fitzgerald's operation in a simple, matter-of-fact manner. Hiding the truth of the operation can make it into a secret and may make the children anxious through fear of the unknown. Trying to hide the scar will lead to all sorts of difficulties, especially as they have always been a very open family. Shutting the children out of the bathroom would create a barrier that had never existed before. Encourage Mr Fitzgerald to bring the children in when his wife is feeling better. This will reassure them that their mother is alright.

9

Possible problem	Advice
Skin irritation	<ul><li>Do not use perfumes, deodorants, soap or talcum powder.</li><li>Always wash the affected area with warm water and pat dry with a soft towel.</li><li>Avoid restrictive clothing and synthetic and coarse materials.</li><li>Expose the area to the air as often as possible.</li><li>Avoid extremes of temperature.</li></ul>
Ink marks showing	<ul><li>Watch out for ink marks. These marks can be washed gently but must not be removed. (The nurse should advise on clothing that will cover the marks.)</li></ul>

Lethargy	• This is normal. Take extra rests in the afternoon and ensure sufficient sleep at night. Refer to a doctor if this is a problem.
	• Encourage your husband and mother-in-law to help.
Anorexia, nausea	• Take small meals regularly. (Good oral hygiene should be encouraged.)
	• Take high-calorie drinks if you are not tolerating food.
	• Refer to a doctor if vomiting occurs.
Stiffness of shoulder	• Continue with exercises you were shown in hospital.
	• Refer to a doctor for physiotherapy.

10
- Support from community staff and the mastectomy nurse
- Attendance at follow-ups, giving time for the discussion of problems
- Fitting of a permanent prosthesis about 6–8 weeks post-operatively
- Counselling agencies—Mastectomy Association, Cancer Help Centre, Cancer Link, British Association for Counselling, and the Women's National Cancer Control Campaign
- Encouragement to resume sports activities, with advice on special clothing, etc.
- Sexual counselling/marriage guidance

3.4 Miss Camerson—a young woman with psoriasis

Anne Camerson is a 22-year-old personal secretary to the sales manager of a pharmaceutical firm. Until recently Anne was engaged to be married to Bob, a police constable. Last month Bob was killed during an armed bank robbery. Anne was distraught and soon afterwards developed widespread circumscribed, dull, reddened skin lesions with flaky silvery scales. Her own family doctor prescribed coal tar ointments with no effect. She has now been admitted for intensive treatment. Dithranol 0.5% in salicylic acid paste has been prescribed.

1 Describe the specific information needed from Anne during her nursing assessment.
2 Anne wants to know what has happened to her skin. How can you explain this?
3 Which one of the following is most likely to have initiated Anne's condition:
   (a) using a different soap?
   (b) distress about her fiancé?
   (c) recent treatment with penicillin?
   (d) contact with a staphylococcal infection?
   Explain the reason for your choice.
4 An introductory course nurse has been assigned to work with you to observe Anne's care. Explain how you would manage this situation.
5 Describe how dithranol acts and the precautions that should be taken when it is used.
6 Anne says that she finds her creams very messy. She has heard of alternative treatments and asks you what these are. How will you reply?
7 One day you find Anne in tears. She says that no-one will find her attractive. How can you help her?
8 What advice should Anne receive on discharge?

3.4   Answers

1

Emotional response The nurse making the assessment will need to know about Anne's response to the lesions and the changes in her appearance. Is anxiety or distress a problem? What is the response of her family and friends? If they are repelled this will upset Anne and will need nursing intervention.

Understanding The nurse will need to find out how much Anne knows about her condition and its treatment. (She may have a close relative with psoriasis and be quite knowledgeable.) Misconceptions or little knowledge will need nursing intervention. Will she be capable of carrying out her own care on discharge?

Socioeconomic factors Does Anne's condition interfere with her work? (For example, nursing is not advisable for someone with a scaly skin condition.) Is her social life affected?

Physical appearance The nurse should pay attention to the appearance and distribution of the lesions. A rough sketch will facilitate evaluation of the treatment. Are there any features of secondary infection? What symptoms is Anne experiencing (e.g. itching, dryness)?

General health The nurse should ask Anne about her nutrition, rest and sleep. If these are upset the added stress may exacerbate her skin condition.

---

2   A good way to start your explanation would be to find out how much Anne knows about the anatomy and physiology of normal skin.

Explain that normally the outer layer of the skin—the epidermis—sheds its surface scales constantly as the scales are rubbed off by friction. The scales that are shed are constantly renewed from below as deep cells multiply and move to the surface, developing into scales as they reach the surface.

In psoriasis, this normal physiology is speeded up and the shedding of scales, which is usually microscopic, becomes obvious.

The cause of psoriasis is not absolutely certain, but it is thought to be an inherited tendency. This tendency may appear as overt lesions during severe emotional or physical trauma.

3 (b). Psoriasis has a known psychological aspect. The other distractors are not specifically related to psoriasis; (a) is more likely to cause contact dermatitis, (c) is related to impetigo, and (d) relates to an allergic skin reaction.

4 First the junior nurse should be taken aside and Anne's condition explained to her (as above). It should be stressed that it is important not to show distaste or to stare at Anne's skin, and that it is not infectious. The junior nurse could be shown a picture of psoriatic lesions in a text-book to prepare her before she meets Anne. She can then be taken to the bedside and introduced to Anne. The care plan can be explained to her and the day's events planned together with Anne.

It is important for Anne's sake that she should be allowed to maintain her modesty during her skin treatment. She should be allowed to bath herself as long as the nurse is within calling distance.

During the skin treatment the junior nurse can be reminded that the creams must be checked from Anne's prescription chart with another nurse. She can be shown how to apply the cream; dithranol should be applied sparingly to the affected skin. Nurses should wear gloves for this procedure as dithranol is harmful to normal skin. (It may be appropriate to explain later that apart from the application of dithranol it is important to touch Anne so that she does not feel unclean or contagious.) A bland starch powder may be dabbed over the dithranol and a tube-gauze suit made to keep the cream in place.

When the treatment is over Anne should be left with something to do. It must be explained to the junior nurse that it is an important part of Anne's treatment to avoid stress, which could be exacerbated by boredom. When the junior nurse has had time to ask any questions away from the bedside, she could return to Anne to talk to her.

5 Dithranol is a keralytic, i.e. it is used to burn away the thickened scales. In doing so, it discolours the skin under the lesions, so the patient should be reassured that this brown discoloration will gradually disappear when the dithranol is discontinued.

The main side-effect of dithranol is erythroderma—a burning sensation and generalized reddening of the skin. For this reason dithranol should be applied sparingly and only to the lesions. Treatment is always commenced with a small percentage of dithranol and the state of the skin assessed before increasing its strength.

6   Anne should be gently told that there is no known cure for psoriasis but that it can usually be controlled in some way. There are other treatments apart from the use of creams but they sometimes have dangerous effects. The policy is always to use local treatments, i.e. creams, first. If Anne does not respond well to these, alternative methods may be considered.

Other methods of treatment are actinotherapy and methotrexate.

(a) **Actinotherapy** This treatment uses ultraviolet light with psoralen tablets, which enhance the body's uptake of treatment. The possible long-term effects of skin cancer have not been fully researched.

(b) **Methotrexate** This is a drug used in cancer to kill rapidly dividing cells. In small doses it can be successful in some patients with psoriasis. The patient has to be carefully monitored as their white cell count can fall dangerously low, and some patients develop cirrhosis of the liver.

7   Find time and privacy to listen to Anne and to discover exactly what are her fears. Touching her arm for reassurance may help Anne to realize that at least the nurse does not find her repulsive.

Anne should be reminded to be patient. Her treatment may be very effective given time. An ex-patient of Anne's age may be invited to come and talk to her. She can also be told about the Psoriasis Association which may help her by sharing common problems.

Anne's friends and relatives should be given an opportunity to talk to the nurse away from the patient. The nurse can explain Anne's fears so that they can also help to reassure her.

8   • **Diet** Avoidance of alcohol in excess is advisable.
    • **Sunlight** Sunbathing is often beneficial provided that the usual protective sun lotions are used.
    • **Stress** Avoidance of stress is advisable. Relaxation methods may be useful. Overwork and overtiredness will also exacerbate her condition and should be avoided.

4 Care of the Sick Child

4.1   Susan Adams—a baby with congenital dislocation of the hip

Susan Adams, aged 6 months, has been admitted to the ward for conservative management of a right dislocated hip. It is planned that management will consist of a period of hoop traction followed by the application of plaster of Paris.

Mr and Mrs Adams have both accompanied Susan to the ward. They are anxious about Susan and at the same time are worried about their other daughter, Claire, aged 2½ years. Mrs Adams would like to be resident but feels guilty about having to leave Claire with friends. Mr Adams is unable to have time off work.

1   What information should the nurse ascertain from Mrs Adams during the initial nursing assessment of Susan?
2   Giving reasons, what advice and support should be given to Mr and Mrs Adams in relation to Claire?

The day after admission, skin traction is applied and Susan's legs are suspended in the perpendicular position for 2 days before gradual abduction is commenced. Hoop traction enables Susan's legs to be abducted, gradually allowing the muscles and ligaments to stretch over a period of time.

3   Describe the specific care Susan will require in relation to her traction.
4   Give an example of the general nursing care Susan will require for a 24-hour period in relation to her activities of living as described by Roper.

Susan's legs continue to be abducted gradually until the position of her legs begins to cause discomfort. Bilateral adductor tenotomies are performed under general anaesthesia from which Susan makes an uneventful recovery. Full abduction is eventually reached 3 weeks after admission and a frog plaster is then applied under a general anaesthetic.

5   Explain the significance of the observations that should be

made when Susan returns from theatre following application of the plaster.

Susan recovers well and is ready for discharge 2 days later.

---

6   What advice and information should be given to Mr and Mrs Adams to enable them to continue Susan's care at home?

During Susan's admission a junior nurse is allocated to you for supervision. She has never looked after a baby with congenital dislocated hips.

---

7   What would you teach the junior nurse about the abnormality and its detection in the neonatal period?
8   The junior nurse asks about Susan's future management. What would be your response?

4.1   Answers

1   The nurse's initial assessment should elicit information about the following:
- Susan's normal activities of living, i.e. her:
  1 normal diet, how much milk she has and what times, what weaning diet she is taking, and any other information
  2 normal elimination pattern and type of nappy worn
  3 normal hygiene routine and any particular soaps/creams used
  4 normal sleep and rest pattern
  5 favourite toys and use of comforters
- her immunization schedule and past infectious diseases
- any known allergies
- her developmental progress and birth weight
- Mr and Mrs Adams' knowledge about Susan's admission and proposed treatment.

2   It is important that Mr and Mrs Adams are not made to feel guilty, whatever they do.

Various researchers have recognized the damaging effects separation may have on a child, particularly on the toddler age group. Claire, at $2\frac{1}{2}$ years, is at a vulnerable age and, even though she is not in hospital, is likely to suffer psychological trauma if separated from her mother. She may well be jealous of Susan since her arrival and this may be aggravated if she is left with friends. As her father is unable to have time off work she would indeed be cut off not only from her parents but also from her normal home environment.

As Mrs Adams feels guilty about leaving Claire with friends it would be best if she did not become resident at the hospital on a permanent basis. There is no reason why she could not bring Claire with her to the hospital and occasionally leave her with friends for short periods of time. The whole family could visit together at the weekends.

Mrs Adams will need support during this period in order that she does not become overtired. Her needs must be met. One nurse must be allocated as Susan's special nurse; this will help Mrs Adams to be more confident about leaving Susan.

3   Susan's buttocks must remain free of the bed as the weight of the child's body provides the countertraction.

Use of benzoin tincture painted onto the skin before extension plasters are applied reduces the risk of allergic reaction and helps the plaster to stick. Crêpe bandages should be removed at least daily to ensure that the plaster is sticking properly. The general condition of the skin should be noted, and exposed areas of the skin washed and dried thoroughly. Check for disturbance of the circulation.

Maintain the position of traction and ensure that abduction is carried out as indicated. Ensure that Susan's feet are warm, and avoid pressure on her heels and ankles. Observe Susan for irritability and crying, which may indicate discomfort.

4

Activity of living	Nursing actions
Personal hygiene and skin care	Give a daily bed bath; change bed linen daily and as necessary; take care of the nappy area—change when the nappy is soiled/wet; be aware of possible areas for the development of pressure sores and keep these areas clean and dry; use sheepskins and observe for signs of pressure.
Eating and drinking	Keep to Susan's normal dietary routine; encourage Mrs Adams to feed Susan when visiting; feed slowly and be aware of the danger of choking; ensure that suction apparatus is available. Record the fluid intake.
Elimination	Potential problems of constipation and urinary infection may develop; ensure adequate fluid intake and record output and bowel functions; observe the urine for signs of infection; send the specimen for analysis if suspect.
Mobility	As mobility is greatly reduced encourage Susan to move and to exercise her unaffected extremities.
Communication	Encourage Mr and Mrs Adams to visit whenever they wish and to bring Claire; spend time talking and playing with Susan; place the cot so that Susan can see what is going on; encourage the parents and nurses to cuddle Susan.

| Play and development | Suspend toys to encourage movement of the arms; provide favourite toys from home and others that will stimulate development: mirrors, peek-a-boo toys, brightly coloured toys, and toys with different textures and sounds. |
| Rest and sleep | Follow the normal pattern where possible; group nursing actions together to allow for sleep and rest periods; give a comforter if one is used. |

5

Observation	Significance
Airway patency	As the anaesthesia is only very light Susan should be fully conscious on return to the ward. She should therefore be able to maintain her own airway.
Respiratory rate and pulse rate, colour, temperature	Observe for any adverse effects of anaesthesia—signs of respiratory depression, tachycardia (may indicate shock), hypothermia. Cyanosis may indicate impending asphyxia.
First passage of urine	Failure to pass urine could indicate retention.
Toes, pedal pulses	Impaired circulation as a result of pressure of the cast may cause discoloration/cyanosis, impaired movement, oedema, temperature changes and absent pedal pulses.

6 All instructions should be given in written form as well as verbally as they are easily forgotten.
  • **Care of the cast** Provide good skin care, paying special attention to the buttocks and groin area. Inspect the skin for signs of irritation; the edges of the cast should be smoothed and covered with waterproof tape. Change nappies as soon as they become soiled. Keep the plaster dry.
  Report any observations that might indicate the formation of a pressure sore, e.g. an offensive odour from the inside of the cast.

Attend the outpatient department as directed for a change of plaster, or earlier if the cast becomes soft or cracked.

- **Positioning and moving Susan** Turn Susan at least every 4 hours. (Instructions should be given on how to turn.) Maintain the correct position of the cast; support Susan with a pillow, allowing her heels to extend beyond the pillow. (Give advice on how to carry Susan and how to secure her in the pram and high chair.)
- **Advice on diet and fluids** Susan should continue with her normal feeds and diet. If she becomes constipated her fluid intake should be increased by giving her extra fluids between feeds.
- **Advice on play and the maintenance of development** Ensure that no small toys can get under the cast. Susan should be stimulated with toys that appeal to the senses and should be encouraged to play on the floor.

Mr and Mrs Adams should be given a date for an outpatient's appointment. Give them the telephone number of the ward and health visitor in case advice is needed. Link them with other families in the same situation. Books and pamphlets are available to help them, e.g. 'Your child in an Immobilising Plaster', an NAWCH publication.

7 First ascertain what the junior nurse already knows about the abnormality. Revise the anatomy of the normal hip joint.

In a congenitally dislocated hip the head of the femur is not within the acetabulum. Without the stimulus of the femoral head the acetabulum fails to develop into a deep socket. The condition is more common in female infants than in male infants.

It is very important that this condition is diagnosed as early as possible so that management can be conservative. Failure to recognize the condition in infancy may prolong treatment, increase the possibility of surgery, and possibly preclude the formation of a normal hip joint.

Screening for hip instability is standard practice and should consist of:

- physical examination for asymmetry of the gluteal folds and apparent shortening of the lower extremity
- testing the degree of abduction with the hip flexed at 90°
- Barlow's test and Ortolani's test (can be demonstrated)

Research is in progress into the detection of instability by recording vibrations created during the above hip tests (Mollan, Bogues and Cowie, *Health Visitor*, August 1983).

8 Susan is likely to stay in plaster for about 6 weeks. X-rays

will then be taken, and if the hips are reduced a splint will be applied, e.g. a Dennis Brown splint, for 6 months to a year. Susan will be seen in the outpatient department at monthly intervals. If the X-rays are not satisfactory, surgery may be necessary.

4.2 Anthony Johnson—an infant with coeliac disease

Anthony Johnson, aged 11 months, has been admitted to the ward for an investigation of his failure to thrive. Anthony gained weight well during the first 4 months of life, but recently began to lose weight. He is now well below his expected weight. Mr and Mrs Johnson are both anxious about Anthony and feel guilty about his weight loss.

Mrs Johnson describes Anthony's stools as pale, fatty and having an offensive odour. On examination Anthony is noted to have abdominal distension and thin arms and legs, and to be a miserable, unhappy baby.

1 What further information does the nurse need about Anthony in order to plan his care?
2 How can the nurse best allay Mr and Mrs Johnson's feelings of guilt?

Various tests are arranged over the next few days including a jejunal biopsy.

3 Describe the nurse's responsibilities in caring for Anthony before, during and after jejunal biopsy.

Coeliac disease is diagnosed following the biopsy and treatment is started immediately.

4 With reference to anatomy and physiology what would you tell the junior nurses on the ward about coeliac disease?
5 What might be your response when Mr and Mrs Johnson ask if treatment will have to be continued throughout his life?

Anthony's treatment consists of dietary regulations and the administration of vitamins.

6 Outline the principles of Anthony's dietary management.
7 What would be the benefits of involving Anthony's parents in his care?

Anthony is ready for discharge 10 days after admission.

8 What advice and help will Mr and Mrs Johnson require to enable them to care for Anthony at home?

4.2 Answers

1

Eating and drinking	(A full dietary history will be taken by a doctor). • What are his likes and dislikes? • What are the normal times of his meals? • What does he drink out of? • Does he like to try to feed himself?
Elimination	• How frequent are his bowel actions? • What type of nappy is he used to? • What types of creams are used on his genital area?
Hygiene	• What is his normal routine for baths and hair washing? • Does he have any particular likes/dislikes at bath time, e.g. toys? • What type of soap/shampoo does Mrs Johnson use for him?
Communication	• Does he have any particular ways of communicating his needs, e.g. pointing, crying, etc.? • How is he consoled if he is upset or miserable?
Sleep	• What are his normal sleep patterns? • What does Mr/Mrs Johnson do if he wakes in the night? • Does he have any special toys for bedtime? • What does he drink before bedtime?
Play	• What are his favourite toys/games? • How does he like to be kept amused? • How well does he play on his own?
Mobility	• Does he pull himself up/crawl? • How well does he get around?
Normal daily routine	• Ask Mrs Johnson to jot down notes about a typical daily routine. A routine helps in making Anthony feel more secure.

Past medical history	• Find out what immunizations he has had and what infections/diseases (if any) he has had.
Family	• Has he any brothers/sisters? If so how old are they and what are their names? • Are there any significant other relatives, e.g. grandparents? • Does Mrs Johnson want to be resident? If not when will she be able to visit?

2
- Be calm, friendly and reassuring towards the family on admission.
- Answer all questions fully.
- Give information about what is happening and keep them fully informed of Anthony's progress at all times.
- Reassure them that Anthony's loss of weight has not been their fault.
- Encourage Mrs Johnson to be resident and to continue to perform all of Anthony's care.
- Encourage them to talk about how they feel, and be available to listen.

3

Preparation for biopsy
- Give an explanation of the procedure to Mrs Johnson.
- Fast Anthony for 4–6 hours before biopsy.
- Administer sedation, e.g. Vallergan as prescribed.
- Allow Anthony to sleep.
- Assist the doctor to pass the capsule.
- Lie Anthony on his right side to aid the passage of the tube.
- Ensure that he does not pull the tube out (restraining him if necessary).
- Take Anthony to the X-ray department. Ensure his safety on route. Lie him on his right side.
- Encourage Anthony's mother to accompany him for his X-ray.

During biopsy
- Hold Anthony if requested by the doctor.
- Talk to Anthony and provide comfort and reassurance.
- Ensure that Anthony is kept warm while he is having his X-ray.
- Comfort Anthony after removal of the capsule.

After biopsy
- Take Anthony back to the ward. Lie him on his side with care—he is still drowsy.
- Once back in his bed, allow him to sleep.
- Inform Mrs Johnson about the procedure.
- Monitor Anthony. You may be requested to take a quarter-hourly pulse rate.
- Encourage Mrs Johnson to feed Anthony when he wakes.

4 Draw a diagram of the intestinal villi (Fig. 11) and explain their role in the absorption of fats, proteins and carbohydrates.

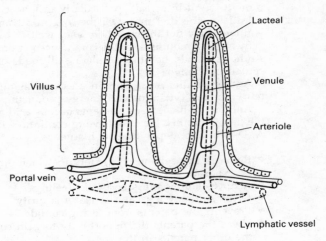

Fig. 11 Villi in the small intestine.

The introduction of dietary gluten into the diet causes atrophy of the intestinal villi, and the lining of the intestine appears flat.

Damage to the mucosa results in malabsorption of fats, proteins and carbohydrates. There is also decreased area for absorption in the bowel. The malabsorption gives rise to signs of failure to thrive.

The causes of coeliac disease are unknown. There does appear to be a familial incidence.

Removal of gluten from the diet will allow the intestinal villi to revert to normal.

5   Ensure that they understand what coeliac disease is and the effects it has on Anthony.

Dietary control will need to be followed throughout life. Stress that Anthony can be perfectly fit and healthy if he continues with a gluten-free diet and that he will lead a normal life.

Research is going on into the management of coeliac disease, and Anthony will be closely monitored.

Some doctors will try a 'gluten challenge' when the children are older to see if they still react unfavourably to the gluten.

6   The basis of dietary treatment of coeliac disease is to exclude all gluten-containing foods from the diet. Gluten is the main protein found in cereals, particularly in wheat and rye.

Initially, the diet may well be low in fat and sugar as Anthony may not tolerate them very well.

By about 2 months after the commencement of treatment, Anthony should be able to tolerate all foods except those containing gluten.

Anthony's diet must contain adequate amounts of protein, minerals, vitamins and energy-producing foods.

Anthony will need supplements of folic acid and iron for the first 2 months. He may have to continue with vitamins A, D, B and C, depending on his needs.

7   • Reduces any separation anxiety to which Anthony will be exposed
     • Reduces family stress and guilt feelings
     • Gives Anthony a greater sense of security
     • Prevents the parents from losing confidence
     • Gives the parents the opportunity to gain comfort from the other parents in the ward
     • Allows the parents to continue in their normal role in being Anthony's main care-givers
     • Improves the rate of recovery
     • Reduces post-hospital reactions

8   • Ensure that they understand what coeliac disease is and how dietary restrictions control the condition.
     • Teach them how to identify those foods that contain gluten (certain products are specially labelled).
     • Arrange for them to spend some time with the dietician, who will give them a list of foods allowed and a list of foods not allowed.
     • Give instructions on how to cope in special circumstances, e.g. going out for meals, parties, etc.

- Teach them about the need for vitamins.
- Teach them about the necessity to continue with the diet, even if Anthony looks and feels well.
- Teach them about the maintenance of good hygiene. Anthony will be prone to infection due to malnutrition and probable anaemia.
- Emotionally upsetting situations may provoke the onset of diarrhoea and coeliac crisis; therefore they should try to maintain a stable environment at home.
- Teach them the signs of coeliac crisis (although this is fairly rare) which are:
  1 severe diarrhoea and vomiting
  2 anorexia
  3 weight
  4 lethargy and immobility
- Tell them what to do if they suspect coeliac crisis (inform the doctor immediately).
- Teach about the importance of regular medical check-ups.
- Put them in touch with the Coeliac Society.

4.3   Phillipa Matthews—a baby with gastroenteritis

Phillipa Matthews, a 6-week-old baby (birth weight 2.8 kg), has been admitted to the ward with a 16-hour history of diarrhoea and vomiting.

Phillipa is the only child of young parents who have recently moved to the area. Mrs Matthews is hoping to return to work as soon as possible as her husband is unemployed and they are experiencing financial difficulties. The family live in a one-bedroomed council flat in a high-rise block. Phillipa is bottle-fed on S.M.A. every 4 hours.

On admission Phillipa is obviously dehydrated with a temperature of 39° C. She has an excoriated bottom and is lethargic. An intravenous infusion is commenced via a scalp vein, and all oral feeding is stopped.

1   With reference to anatomy and physiology explain why Phillipa has become dehydrated so quickly and the possible effects of fluid and electrolyte loss.

2   What information would it be important to ascertain from Mrs Matthews during the initial nursing assessment?

3   Explain the significance of the observations of Phillipa on admission and during the first 24 hours.

4   The priority of Phillipa's management is to replace lost fluid and electrolytes. Identify the potential problems associated with the administration of intravenous fluids to Phillipa and outline the nursing actions you might implement to prevent/direct these problems.

5   Explain, giving reasons, the precautions the nurse should take to prevent the spread of infection to other young children.

6   List some other problems (actual or potential) Phillipa may have on admission.

48 hours after admission oral fluids are reintroduced and the intravenous infusion is reduced accordingly.

7   Discuss the principles involved in the regrading of Phillipa's feeds.

8   Calculate the amount of feed Phillipa will require every 24 hours once she is back to normal feeds.

Phillipa's mother is extremely anxious and concerned about her baby and admits to being unsure of how to care for her. She is worried about taking her home since she has no-one on whom she may call for help. Mr Matthews does not appear to give his wife very much support.

---

9   In preparing the family for discharge what should Mr and Mrs Matthews be taught regarding:
   (a) the prevention of further bouts of diarrhoea?
   (b) feeding and baby hygiene?
   (c) how to meet Phillipa's developmental needs?

10   How can the effectiveness of Phillipa's care be evaluated when she is ready for discharge 6 days after admission?

11   Identify the help and support that is available in the community for Mr and Mrs Matthews. Describe the nurses' role in arranging the provision of this help before discharge.

4.3   Answers

1   Phillipa has become dehydrated quickly for the following reasons:
   - Infants have relatively small nutritional reserves.
   - Seventy to eighty per cent of their body weight is water (compared with 60% of body weight in adults).
   - In comparison with adults infants have a greater percentage of body water in their extracellular compartment.
   - The turnover of water is much greater in infants than in adults:
      1 The metabolic rate is higher.
      2 There is a greater body surface area in relation to weight.
      3 The immature kidney is unable to conserve water.
   - Young infants cannot independently respond to excessive loss by adapting their intake.

   Dehydration may be hypotonic, isotonic or hypertonic depending on the electrolytes lost. Metabolic acidosis may develop due to loss of potassium and bicarbonate in the stools. The effects on the baby depend on the degree of dehydration, as follows:
   - **Mild dehydration** This results in 2½–5% body weight loss, leading to dry skin and mucous membranes, poor skin turgor, crying and irritability.
   - **Moderate dehydration** This results in 5–10% body weight loss, leading to the above features plus a depressed anterior fontanelle, irritability/lethargy, sunken eyes and reduced urine output.
   - **Severe dehydration** This results in more than 10% body weight loss, leading to limpness, apathy, tachycardia, tachypnoea, cold extremities, weak peripheral pulses and oliguria.

2   Much information can be gained later but the following facts will be needed immediately:
   - whether Phillipa's mother is resident or non-resident. If non-resident a telephone number is needed for contact together with a contact number for the father.
   - Phillipa's weight before this illness.
   - a brief description from Phillipa's mother of the illness and a description of Phillipa's normal behaviour.
   - her normal nutritional requirements. At what times is she usually fed? Does she have a dummy/comforter?

- her normal elimination habits. What barrier cream/nappy is normally used?
- her sleeping habits. What position does she prefer for resting?

3

Observation	Significance
Weight (expected weight 3.6 kg)	A comparison of the actual weight with the weight before the illness gives the doctor an indication of the degree of hydration and a basis for fluid administration.
Pulse (average normal=120 beats/min)	A rapid, weak pulse indicates dehydration and sodium excess; a bounding pulse, not easily obliterated, indicates a fluid volume excess due to an over-administration of intravenous fluids.
Respiration (average normal=30–35 respirations/min)	Rapid, deep respirations indicate metabolic acidosis; slow, shallow respirations indicate respiratory alkalosis; dyspnoea indicates fluid volume excess.
Temperature (normal=37° C)	The temperature indicates the degree of pyrexia and the need for intervention.
Skin	Cold extremities indicate severe fluid volume and sodium loss; the degree of turgor indicates the degree of dehydration.
Behaviour	Hypotonia indicates a potassium deficit; weakness indicates metabolic acidosis; lethargy/irritability indicates a fluid volume deficit.

4

Problem	Nursing actions
As only small amounts are being given: • it can be difficult to regulate • there is a danger of overhydration	• Use a paediatric giving set with a graduated burette. • Use an infusion pump—DANGER—pumps will continue to work against resistance when the needle is out of the vein.

The cannula can become easily dislodged as:
- the baby's veins are small and friable
- an active baby may pull on the cannula tubing

Long lengths of intravenous tubing are dangerous as the tubing can strangle a baby if it is left hanging in the cot/crib.

The mother may be frightened to nurse the baby with an infusion.

- Observe the pulse/respiration and the intake/output.
- Appropriate restraint should be applied, i.e. not too tight and the needle should be visible.
- Check the site for swelling and redness hourly.

- Ensure that any long lengths of tubing are tied out of baby's reach.
- Instruct the mother to observe the tubing for any danger.
- Explain the purpose of the infusion.
- Show the mother how to pick Phillipa up and hold her without dislodging the needle.
- Involve the mother in observing the fluid level in the burette and any swelling around the needle site.

5   Precautions may depend upon local hospital policies, so refer to these as needed.
- Isolate Phillipa in a cubicle with hand-washing facilities including soap dispensers.
- Hand washing. Washing the hands after touching Phillipa and her equipment removes harmful organisms if done *efficiently*. Taps should be elbow operated.
- Use gowns and gloves as hospital policy requires. A disposable plastic gown should be worn under a white cotton gown as cotton gowns are ineffective against bacteria when wet. Gloves reduce contamination of the hands.
- Correctly dispose of waste, infected linen and nappies according to hospital policy.
- Phillipa's own equipment should be kept in the cubicle; this prevents sharing it with other children.
- Give careful explanations to Phillipa's mother and father. Reduce visitors as much as possible (no children).
- Put a notice on the cubicle door to inform *all* staff of the precautions to be taken.
- Staff allocated to care for Phillipa should be kept to a minimum.
- Toys used by Phillipa should be washable.

- The cubicle should be cleaned according to the policy on discharge.
- A nurse should be allocated to Phillipa to avoid contact with other patients who may be put at risk.

6 Phillipa is likely to have some of the following problems:
- potential inhalation of vomit
- a dry mouth, with possible thrush
- excoriated buttocks
- pyrexia
- dehydration
- frequent loose, explosive stools

7 Phillipa's readiness to recommence oral feeds will be assessed by:
- her state of hydration
- improvement of diarrhoea
- cessation of vomiting

First feeds should be a glucose/electrolyte solution given in small amounts 3-hourly.

Milk feeds should be introduced gradually over the next 24–48 hours beginning with quarter strength milk. Build up the strength slowly to allow toleration.

If Phillipa has any more vomiting or diarrhoea she may have to have further clear feeds.

8 Phillipa should be fed according to her expected weight. Babies gain approximately 200 grams per week for the first 3 months of life (disregarding the first 2 weeks during which time they lose weight).

Phillipa should therefore have gained 200 g × 4 = 800 g (0.8 kg)

∴ Expected weight = birth weight (2.8 kg) + 0.8 kg = **3.6 kg**.

The fluid requirement for a full-term infant is 150 ml/kg/day

∴ Phillipa's fluid requirement = 3.6 × 150 ml/day = **540 ml/day**.

9 (a) Ensure correct preparation of feeds, handling and storage of equipment, and correct methods of sterilization. Make sure to wash hands, particularly after changing nappies. Dummies should be sterilized if used. Mr and Mrs Matthews should know what to do if she develops diarrhoea again.

(b) Mr and Mrs Matthews should know how to calculate the amount of feed Phillipa requires and how to make up the formula correctly, and what to give her if she's thirsty/appears hungry in between feeds. Watch Mr/Mrs Matthews bath Phillipa, and give advice about hygiene and care of the nappy area.

(c) Talk to both parents about what to expect from Phillipa

over the next few weeks. Tell them what toys are best to stimulate Phillipa, giving them ideas for inexpensive toys. Stress the importance of talking to Phillipa, spending time touching her and making eye contact. Small babies often enjoy soft music. Give some written advice.

10
- Stools are improved in colour, content and consistency of faeces, and reduced in frequency.
- There is no vomiting.
- Her pulse, respirations and temperature lie within the normal limits.
- Her skin turgor is normal, with no signs of dehydration.
- She is tolerating normal feeds well.
- Her nappy area is healed (or healing well).
- She has gained weight.
- She is a relaxed, rested and contented baby.
- Her parents understand the advice given and are happy to go home.

11
- The health visitor must be informed of Phillipa's discharge. She will arrange a home visit beforehand to monitor conditions, and will make regular visits after Phillipa's return home. She will advise and provide support regarding feeding, hygiene, development and any other problems regarding child care.
- The general practitioner will be informed of Phillipa's discharge.
- Contact should be made with the social worker before discharge. Help can be given with financial difficulties and employment.
- The local baby clinic will enable Mrs Matthews to mix with other young mothers and make some friends.
- Local support groups exist to help Mr and Mrs Matthews.

4.4   Gillian Simpson—a toddler who has been the victim of non-accidental injury

Gillian, aged 18 months, is the youngest of Mr and Mrs Simpson's three children. She has a sister aged 2½ years and a brother aged 4 years. The family live in a two-bedroomed eighth floor flat in the middle of a large housing estate. They have only recently moved there and have no relatives nearby. Mr Simpson works very long hours to earn extra money.

Mrs Simpson has brought Gillian to the accident and emergency department on four occasions recently for no apparent reason. On this occasion Mr Simpson has brought Gillian explaining that she had fallen and bumped herself on a hot radiator.

On examination the following are noted:
- a number of bruises of different ages over Gillian's body
- a swollen, painful left arm
- small burn marks on her feet and buttocks
- extensive nappy rash

As non-accidental injury is suspected, Gillian is to be admitted to the children's ward. Mr Simpson becomes angry and refuses to allow Gillian to be admitted. The hospital social worker is contacted and the decision made to obtain a 'place of safety order'.

1   How is a 'place of safety' order obtained and who issues it?
2   Outline the nursing care Gillian will require in order to meet her needs while she is in hospital.
3   What actions would you take when Mr and Mrs Simpson arrive the following day and insist on taking Gillian home?

A detailed examination of Gillian is carried out, including X-rays that indicate a number of old fractures. A case conference is hastily arranged.

4   List the personnel who should be present at the case conference.
5   What will be the purpose of the case conference?

A few days after Gillian has been admitted Mrs Simpson breaks down and admits to having abused Gillian.

6　Discuss the factors that may have predisposed to Mrs Simpson's behaviour.

7　What attitudes should the nurse demonstrate in order to encourage Mrs Simpson to talk about what has happened?

8　What are the alternative outcomes of the case conference?

4.4   Answers

1   The Social Services Department or NSPCC can obtain a removal order ('place of safety order') from any magistrate's court during the day or from a Justice of the Peace out of hours. This order allows the child to be kept in a 'place for safety' for a maximum period of 28 days.

In extreme emergencies the police may grant an 8-day 'place of safety order'. They do not need to go to a Justice of the Peace or a magistrate's court.

2

Need	Nursing actions
To form trusting relationships	• Assign one nurse to care for Gillian for the majority of the time. • Touch Gillian gently. • Provide non-threatening contact, e.g. cuddling. • Set limits for her and be consistent. • Be honest. • Utilize a 'granny scheme' if one is available.
To be safe	Under a 'place of safety order' parents are not allowed to remove Gillian from the hospital. • Revise your knowledge of developmental progress of 18-month-old children in order to ensure a safe environment for Gillian.
To satisfy physiological needs (hunger and thirst)	• Revise your basic knowledge of dietary requirements of 18-month-old children. • Provide food that she likes. • Don't force her to eat. • Give fluids—find out the words she uses and the drinks she likes. • Ascertain how she normally eats and what she drinks out of.
To keep her warm	• Dress her in suitable clothes.
To ensure good elimination habits	• Ensure that her nappy is changed whenever it is wet. • Apply cream to any nappy rash and leave it exposed when possible. • Don't try to begin potty training.

To ensure cleanliness	• Find out her normal routine and follow it as much as possible, but ensure regular baths and hand and face washes, and teeth cleaning every morning and evening. • Hair should be washed as required. • Nails should be trimmed as required.
To ensure adequate rest and sleep	• Follow her normal routine regarding any afternoon naps. • Follow her usual bedtime routines and ensure that she has an adequate night's sleep.
To develop motor skills and language skills	• Provide opportunities for different types of play, e.g. energetic, creative and skilful play. • Use toys that appeal to the senses and introduce 'messy' play. • Provide a stimulating environment. • Talk to Gillian and find out any special words that she uses. • Integrate Gillian with other children for play activities, meal-times, etc.

3 • Explain to the parents that they are not in authority to remove Gillian and find out if they understand about the 'place of safety order'.
  • Allocate a nurse to stay with Gillian.
  • If the parents still insist on removing Gillian, inform a social worker/consultant.
  • If you have difficulty with the parents, inform the security personnel and/or the porters for assistance.
  • Try to keep all arguments and discussions away from Gillian, i.e. in Sister's office.
  • As a last resort, the police may have to be informed.

4 • Social worker
  • Paediatric consultant
  • General practitioner
  • Medical officer
  • Health visitor
  • NSPCC representative
  • Police officer
  • Head teacher of day nursery/nursery centre
  • Ward Sister

5   • To share knowledge of and concern about the family
      • To formulate a diagnosis and full family assessment
      • To decide on whether or not to recommend registration
      • To formulate a treatment plan and long-term aims
      • To allocate responsibilities for the implementation of plans
      • To decide whether or not to inform the parents of registration
      • To nominate a key worker
      • To decide on ongoing procedure

6   Discussion should cover the following points:
      • Mrs Simpson's background—possible abuse in childhood, quality of care during childhood, feelings and emotional states, size of family, economic conditions of family
      • Isolation from the extended family and from friends (on her own with three small children for much of the day)
      • Tension in the family possibly caused by lack of money, three small children, marital disharmony, and the difficulty of living with small children in a high rise block of flats
      • Views on discipline
      • The behaviour of the child, which may provoke abuse
      • Feelings of inadequacy, low self-esteem, and fear of rejection

7   • Assume a non-judgemental attitude.
      • Do not be threatening.
      • Do not ask questions about the incident.
      • Listen to what she says.
      • Do not challenge any information she may give.
      • Serve as a role model in the management of Gillian and her behaviour.
      • Express appropriate care and concern.
      • Stay objective but be empathetic.
      • Endeavour to come to terms with your own feelings of anger and contempt.

8   A decision will be reached as to whether or not to place Gillian's name on the 'at risk register'.
    The main aim of management is to rehabilitate the family and keep them together. This may involve:
      • day care
      • mothers groups
      • psychotherapy
      • help with the social/economic situation
      • short-term residential care

- voluntary supervision
- fostering

Legal action may be taken in that the parents may be prosecuted. This may result in prison sentences, or probation. Gillian may be removed to permanent foster care.

The Magistrate's Court/Crown Court gives criminal proceedings; the Juvenile Court gives Care Proceedings.

4.5 Michael Davies—a baby with congenital hypertrophic pyloric stenosis

Michael Davies, aged 6 weeks, has been admitted to the ward with suspected congenital hypertrophic pyloric stenosis. He is accompanied by both his parents who are extremely anxious about him. He is their first baby and they had been trying for a baby for 2 years.

Mr Davies has recently been made redundant and is finding it difficult to get alternative employment. The family live in a two-bedroomed, newly built town house. Neither have relatives living in the area.

Michael has been vomiting on and off for 2 weeks but over the past 2 days the vomiting has become more persistent. He is now vomiting after every feed. The vomit is projectile and contains milk curds and blood. Michael looks anxious and has lost weight. He is moderately dehydrated.

Mrs Davies had been breast-feeding Michael for the first 3 weeks of life but had decided to change to bottle-feeding.

1. Explain the significance of the above information gained during an initial nursing assessment.
2. Describe the nurse's role during a test feed, which the doctor asks to be carried out shortly after admission.
3. Identify the ways in which the nursing staff may reduce Mr and Mrs Davies' anxiety.
4. What would you tell a junior colleague about the reasons for Michael's problems?

Following confirmation of the diagnosis, surgery is planned for about 5 hours time. A nasogastric tube is passed and an intravenous infusion is commenced to restore the fluid and electrolyte balance. A gastric lavage is to be performed as part of Michael's pre-operative preparation.

5. Identify, giving reasons, the steps you would take to ensure that the gastric lavage is carried out safely.

Michael returns to the ward following a pyloromyotomy under general anaesthetic. He is conscious on return to the ward.

6   Explain the significance of the post-operative observations you would make on Michael.

7   Discuss the principles of the reintroduction of milk feeds following surgery.

During Michael's stay Mr and Mrs Davies admit to being very unsure of the most suitable toys to buy for him.

8   With reference to normal growth and development what advice would you give them?

9   What arrangements should be made before Michael is discharged home 4 days later?

4.5 Answers

1

Information	Significance
Michael is 6 weeks old.	This gives an indication of his developmental stage, and of his needs while in hospital. Because of his immature immune system he may pick up hospital infection, so he should be nursed in a cubicle with protective precautions.
	Age also indicates that parents will still be building up a bond with him and need to be encouraged to continue this.
He is the first baby after 2 years of trying.	This is liable to make them more anxious and frightened of losing Michael. They may feel guilty and that they have caused his illness.
Mr Davies is redundant and they live in a new town house.	They may well have financial problems as they are likely to have a fairly high mortgage.
They have no relatives living in the area.	They may well feel isolated and lacking in support from parents.
Michael has projectile vomiting, looks anxious, is dehydrated, and has lost weight.	This is indicative of pyloric stenosis.
Mrs Davies has recently changed from breast-feeding to bottle-feeding.	She may feel that Michael's illness is all her fault caused by the discontinuation of breast-feeding.

2 The purpose of the test feed is for the doctor to be able to confirm the diagnosis by:
   1 the presence of visible peristalsis
   2 palpation of the thickened pylorus muscle
   The nurse must ensure that Michael is warm and comfortable and that he lies with his abdomen exposed to allow

the doctor to observe for peristalsis. The doctor may well ask for Michael to be given his normal feed to ensure that he takes it. It would be much better for Michael's mum to feed him, and the nurse should explain what to do and why it is being done. Following the test feed ensure that if Michael vomits his airway is maintained.

3
- Greet Mr and Mrs Davies calmly on admission. Offer them a seat in Michael's cubicle and a cup of tea.
- Introduce yourself and ask them about Michael and his normal routine.
- Explain all procedures as they are performed.
- Ensure that they understand what the doctor has told them.
- Involve them in Michael's care, e.g. with the test feed.
- Offer Mrs Davies residency. Mr Davies may well wish to stay also.
- Reassure them that they are in no way to blame for what has happened to Michael and that the change from breast- to bottle-feeding would not have caused it.
- Enlist the help of the social worker if they have financial worries, e.g. travelling costs.

4   Ascertain what the student nurse already knows about pyloric stenosis.

With the use of a diagram explain the position of the pylorus and the effect of a thickened muscle at this sphincter.

The thickened muscle blocks the outlet from the stomach. As the muscle thickens so the degree of obstruction increases. This accounts for the developing frequency and force of the vomiting.

The muscles of the stomach contract strongly to attempt to overcome the obstruction, giving rise to visible peristalsis.

Eventually the vomiting becomes projectile, the force of which comes from the strong muscular contractions in the stomach.

The vomitus contains milk curds, mucus and blood. The blood arises from irritation of the lining of the oesophagus by hydrochloric acid.

As no milk is passing on into the bowel, Michael will be constipated or will have decreased frequency bowel movements.

With continued vomiting Michael becomes quickly dehydrated. In particular he loses potassium, leading to metabolic acidosis.

A lack of milk leads to weight loss and a hungry, anxious baby.

5

Action	Reasons
Withdraw some fluid using a syringe, and check the aspirate with litmus paper.	It is important to ensure that the tube is in the stomach. Stomach contents are acid and will turn the blue litmus paper red.
Use no more than 90 ml of fluid.	This prevents overdistension of the stomach.
Measure all fluid returned.	This ensures complete emptying of the stomach and helps maintenance of an intake and output chart.
Use only normal saline (at a temperature of 37° C).	Only isotonic fluids must be used. Using water can lead to water intoxication.
Enlist the help of another nurse/mother to maintain Michael in a lateral position.	This minimizes the risk of inhalation of vomit during the lavage.

6

Observation	Significance
Hourly measurement of pulse rate/apex beat	The normal pulse rate at this age is 120–140 beats/min. An increase could indicate shock, haemorrhage or pain.
Half-hourly respiration rate	The normal rate is 30–40 respirations per minute. An irregular rate may be indicative of acidosis. A raised rate may indicate respiratory difficulty.
Blood pressure on return from theatre (repeated only if unstable)	Normal blood pressure at this age is about 75/50 mmHg. This is difficult to determine and should be done with an electronic device. A lower than normal blood pressure reading may mean shock/haemorrhage, but is a late sign.

Colour and general behaviour	Cyanosis may indicate respiratory difficulty. Anxiety and/or restlessness may be indicative of pain.
Observation of the wound site at regular intervals	Watch for any signs of oozing or haemorrhage.
Intake and output chart	Failure to pass urine within 12 hours of surgery should be reported to doctors as it may indicate retention. Input from an intravenous infusion may be over/under-infusing.
	Any vomiting may indicate perforation of the bowel at the time of operation, as may increased nasogastric tube aspirate.
Parents' reaction to Michael	This gives an idea of how they are coping with Michael's illness and the degree to which they are meeting their own needs.

7 Oral feeds can be reintroduced 2–4 hours following surgery depending on Michael's condition. As oral feeding increases, so the rate of the infusion will be decreased. The nasogastric tube is secured initially by means of a spigot and then removed when feeding is established.

Different hospitals have different post-operative feeding regimens but the principles are the same.

The quantity of fluid given is increased slowly to give the pylorus muscle time to expand.

The first few feeds are usually dextrose/saline and then slowly graduated back to full strength milk. The strength of the milk is increased before the quantity is increased.

Some areas go back a step in the regimen if vomiting occurs. Whatever the policy, all vomiting should be recorded and its characteristics noted.

The main aim of the reintroduction of feeds is to have Michael back on his normal feeds within 48–72 hours.

8 Explain that development is a very individual thing and that each child develops at his own rate. At Michael's stage of development:

- he will be able to momentarily fixate visually on an object or a human face

- he will be able to follow bright moving objects from side to side and up and down
- he will immediately drop any objects placed in his hands
- he will respond to noises, e.g. bells, and to the human voice
- he will show interest in the human face and may have begun to smile
- responses are normally limited to discomfort
- he will enjoy sucking and being held, cuddled and rocked

Taking this into consideration Mr and Mrs Davies can be advised to:

- use the human face (by smiling at Michael and talking to him)
- hold, touch, kiss and cuddle him
- call him by his name
- play soft music and sing to him
- dangle bright, moving objects in his field of vision
- explain how to make safe mobiles out of household items
- expose him to different sounds around the house
- play with him when he is awake
- use brightly-coloured linen and clothing

9 Any problems with finance should be investigated by the social worker.

The health visitor should be contacted and should have organized a pre-discharge home visit to ensure that the family have all they need.

A letter should be sent to the Davies' general practitioner.

Information regarding Michael's care and wound should be given to Mr and Mrs Davies. If stitches need to be removed the district nurse must be contacted.

An outpatient's appointment should be made.

Transport arrangements should be checked.

4.6 Alison Boycott—a pre-school child having a tonsillectomy

Alison Boycott, aged 4 years, has been admitted to the ward for tonsillectomy. She is accompanied by her mother who wishes to be resident.

Alison was born at term by normal delivery and has progressed well, walking at 13 months and gaining bladder and bowel control by the age of 2½ years. She has been attending the local play-group since she was 3 and is to start infant school in 8 months time. She has two older brothers who are both fit and well.

Her mother works as a part-time dental receptionist and her father is a salesman.

1   With reference to some of the relevant research, why is the preparation of children for hospital so important and how may Mr and Mrs Boycott have been helped to prepare Alison for the admission?

2   Explain the significance of the above information concerning Alison and her family during the initial assessment.

3   Identify the additional information required in order to plan Alison's care.

4   With reference to normal growth and development explain how Alison's needs can be met with regard to:
   (a) psychological preparation for theatre
   (b) maintenance of a safe environment
   (c) play

5   Explain the importance of family-centred care and describe how Alison's family should be involved during her stay in hospital.

6   As part of her pre-operative preparation Alison is prescribed trimeprazine (Vallergan) 51 mg. How much should she be given from a stock solution of 30 mg in 5 ml? What may be the side-effects of this drug?

On the day of operation Alison goes to theatre at 9.30 a.m. She returns from theatre having regained consciousness in the recovery room.

7   What post-operative observations would be carried out and what would be their significance?

8 Explain, giving reasons, the specific complications that might occur following Alison's surgery.

Four hours post-operatively Alison shows signs of haemorrhage and suddenly vomits 200 ml of fresh blood. Her mother, who is with her, faints. Alison begins to cry and feels sick again.

---

9 Select five items from the following list of possible actions and, giving reasons, place them in order of priority to show how the nurse should manage this situation. (Actions may be grouped together if priority is difficult to judge.)
- Administer oxygen to Alison.
- Apply ice to the bridge of Alison's nose.
- Stay with Alison and reassure her.
- Prepare mother and child for the possibility of return to theatre.
- Give Mrs Boycott a drink of water and sit her in a chair.
- Continue monitoring Alison's pulse and respirations quarter-hourly.
- Sit Alison upright with a vomit bowl.
- Clean the blood away from Alison's face.
- Call for assistance from a senior member of staff.
- Ask somebody to.attend to Mrs Boycott.
- Loosen Mrs Boycott's collar.

10 Prepare written instructions for Mr and Mrs Boycott to take with them on discharge to enable them to continue Alison's care at home.

4.6   Answers

1   The most well-known research includes:
Eiser, C. & Patterson D. (1984) Children's perceptions of hospital—a preliminary study. *International Journal of Nursing Studies* Vol. 21, No. 1.
Harris, P.J. (1981) Preparation of parents and their children for a planned hospital admission. *Nursing Times* Oct. 7.
Rodin, J. (1983) *'Will this hurt?'* London: Royal College of Nursing
Stewart, A. (1984) Prepared for parting. *Nursing Mirror* Vol. 159, No. 17.
These pieces of research all come to the conclusion that the preparation of children reduces stress and increases the child's well-being in hospital. It also reduces the parents' anxiety, which is good for the child.

Preparation must be geared to the individual child, with his age, past experience and personality being taken into account.

Mr and Mrs Boycott should have been spoken to before Alison's admission and given information regarding:
- practical details—length of stay, requirements, residence
- medical details—an explanation about tonsils, what the operation involves, and what to expect before and after the operation
- hospital routine
- how to expect Alison to react
- ideas about how to prepare Alison—books to read; games and toys about hospital; to be honest; to arrange a visit to the hospital; help in buying new pyjamas, etc; how to explain separation from the family and how to answer Alison's questions.

Written advice should also have been given.

2

Information	Significance
Alison is 4 years old.	This enables the nurse to be able to give care based on the needs of this particular age group.
Her mother wishes to be resident.	Her mother will therefore be able to be with Alison throughout her stay, and care can be planned around this fact.

Alison had a normal term delivery and has developed normally.	This informs the nurse that Alison is progressing at an average rate.
Alison has bladder and bowel control.	This informs the nurse of what to expect from Alison and that any accidents are a sign of regression.
Alison has been attending the local play-group.	This indicates that Alison is used to being with other children and being away from her mother for short periods of time.
Alison has two older brothers.	Alison will be used to the company of her brothers. They will have influenced her development and are an important part of her life. They are both at school, so will need looking after out of school hours.
Mrs Boycott works part time as a dental receptionist.	She may well have had some kind of training and may be quite capable of understanding an involved explanation, but the nurse should avoid use of jargon and realize that she may not be familiar with hospitals.
Alison's father is a salesman.	He may therefore be away from home for periods of time, so he may not be available to look after the boys.

3   Information is needed about:
   - any previous hospital admissions
   - what she has been told about the forthcoming surgery
   - her normal daily routine
   - eating and drinking—her likes and dislikes (especially drinks), her usual pattern of eating, and the ability to feed herself
   - communication—language development and any special words
   - hygiene—her normal routine, ability to take care of her own hygiene and dressing, and ability to clean her own teeth
   - sleep routine—use of a night light, time she goes to bed, any special routine before bed, whether she wakes up at night, use of a comforter
   - play—favourite toys and games
   - immunization programme—any infectious diseases she has had
   - normal elimination pattern—special words for toilet
   - recent colds or sore throats

4   (a) Pre-school children see the world from their own view-
point. They have a great fear of bodily injury and mutilation.
They have an inability to understand in several dimensions
and do not usually comprehend degrees of ill and good.
They understand the concept of time in the present and to
some extent in the past, but have limited comprehension of
'the future'. Pre-schoolers need visual aids in order for them
to understand a concept.

The following knowledge can be used in preparing Alison
for theatre:

- Use concrete terms and visual aids to describe procedure,
  i.e. gowns, masks, syringes and any other equipment that
  may be used. Be honest.
- Utilize a favourite doll to demonstrate the procedure;
  role-play should be encouraged as it allows emotions to
  be dealt with.
- Introduce anxiety-laden information as the last item.
- Involve the mother in explanations.
- Stress the positive effects of the operation. For example,
  'When your tonsils are fixed you won't have as many
  sore throats'.
- When explaining the timing of events, use other measur-
  able indicators, e.g. bedtime, meal-times, the time play-
  group ends.
- Evaluate explanations, e.g. by watching Alison play to
  highlight any misconceptions.

(b) Pre-schoolers are very active and inquisitive, with
developing self-control but an immature understanding of
danger. For example:

- They can reach door-knobs and are eager to explore.
- They enjoy taking things apart, putting them together
  and experimenting.
- They are nimble on their feet and often in a hurry.
- They are capable of taking verbal instructions and learn-
  ing simple safety routines.

Actions that the nurse can take in relation to the above
are as follows:

- Door-knobs should be out of reach and doors kept shut,
  especially doors to the sluice, bathroom, kitchen and
  treatment room.
- Dangerous items, e.g. electrical equipment, must be kept
  out of reach where possible, and wires should not be
  trailing.
- Alison should not be allowed to run about with anything

in her mouth, e.g. spoons, or holding pens/pencils.
- Alison should wear her slippers when out of bed.
- Toys and the play area should be safe.
- Explain reasons for out-of-bound areas and things she is not allowed to do.

(c) Children do regress to some extent in hospital and often like to play with toys long forgotten. Explain this to parents so that they understand.

It is important to assess Alison's individual needs regarding play, i.e. what she likes to play with and what she is able to do. Toys must be kept safe.

Pre-school children generally enjoy:
- group play, and are capable of simple interactive play
- games that allow for creativity, e.g. drawing and painting
- being read to
- physical games when well

When Alison has had surgery she will need quieter forms of play but can still interact with other children. Her mother will be able to keep her occupied.

5 Alison belongs to her family and they are all important to her. She needs to have continued contact with all members of her family including grandparents to maintain a sense of security. It is the family who know best how to care for Alison.

The family may feel frustrated if they cannot contribute to Alison's care; mother especially may feel inadequate/guilty about the suffering her daughter is having to cope with. Father may feel left out, especially if a hospital admission is a long one. It is important for parents to be allowed to remain with their child because they provide emotional support.

Siblings may feel forgotten or left out. They may feel that they have done something wrong to make their sister ill and their imagination may run away with them. Visiting Alison will help her brothers overcome any misconceptions.

Involve the parents as much as they wish and form a good working relationship. Discuss Alison's care together with them to ensure that the best actions are taken. Listen to Alison's mother's reports on Alison. Teach Mrs Boycott where necessary. Give her the option of being present during procedures. Ensure that she gets her meals and a break away from the ward. Encourage free visiting for all members of the family.

6   The formula to use to work out the dosage required is as follows:

$$\frac{\text{What you want}}{\text{What you've got}} \times \text{dilution (ml)}$$

$$= \frac{51}{30} \times 5$$

$$= \frac{51}{6} = 8.5 \text{ ml}$$

The side-effects of trimeprazine are minimal. Some children may develop tremor, excitability and insomnia. Atropine-like effects include a dry mouth, fever and rash, and an overdosage may cause hallucinations, coma and convulsions. Trimeprazine will increase the effects of other drugs such as anticonvulsants and may cause hypotension.

7

Observation	Significance
Pulse	An increasing rapid pulse is indicative of haemorrhage.
Respiratory rate	An increased respiratory rate may indicate increasing respiratory difficulty.
Degree of swallowing	Frequent swallowing is indicative of haemorrhage.
Colour	Pallor is a sign that Alison may be bleeding. Cyanosis indicates respiratory difficulty.
Behaviour	Restlessness is indicative of haemorrhage.
Vomiting	Fresh blood is indicative of haemorrhage. Alison may vomit old blood initially.
Temperature	A rise in temperature is indicative of infection

8

Complication	Reason
Primary haemorrhage	This occurs at the time of operation or within a few hours due to a slipped ligature.

Reactionary haemorrhage	This occurs within the first 12–24 hours after surgery due to the blood pressure returning to normal following anaesthesia.
Secondary haemorrhage	This occurs 2–10 days following surgery and is due to infection at the site of the tonsil bed. The infection erodes blood vessels.
Infection	This may occur if Alison is reluctant to drink and eat following surgery, and can predispose to secondary haemorrhage.

9 It is appreciated that priority questions may be difficult to answer. However, in this circumstance the nurse should take certain actions as follows:

Action	Rationale
Sit Alison upright with a vomit bowl, stay with her and reassure her.	This ensures that a clear airway is maintained. Alison is conscious enough to automatically wish to sit up as she vomits. It is essential to stay with Alison.
Call for assistance from a senior member of staff.	Help must be sought almost immediately in order to: • gain advice regarding further actions • inform the surgeon urgently • assist and reassure Mrs Boycott
Continue to monitor Alison's pulse and respiratory rate	This assesses the degree of haemorrhage and shock. The pulse may become more rapid and difficult to palpate, irregularities may occur, and respirations are increased and shallow if the shock becomes more severe.
Clear blood away from Alison's face.	This makes Alison more comfortable.
Prepare Alison and her mother for possible return to theatre.	Alison will be returned to theatre as soon as possible, so Mrs Boycott (when recovered) and Alison must be told.

10 It is important to give written instructions to back up verbal advice as parents often forget what they have been told. Written information should include:
• **instructions about diet and fluids**. A normal diet should be encouraged to prevent infection by encouraging mus-

cular activity and preventing the formation of slough. Fluids will also help to keep the area clean.

- **rest and sleep**. Alison may need an afternoon nap initially and an early night. Alison should be encouraged to play in the fresh air.
- **advice about analgesia**. This should be given as prescribed before meals if Alison complains of pain on swallowing. Any persistent problems should be reported to their general practitioner.
- **no school** until after an ear, nose and throat appointment. A date should be given for this appointment. Alison should avoid swimming.
- **advice to avoid crowded places**, e.g. shops, while infection is more likely to be contracted.
- **bleeding**. If any bleeding occurs, or they are worried about Alison, they must contact their general practitioner or hospital.

5 Care of the Patient with Problems of the Nervous System

5.1   Janice Bagnall—a young girl with epilepsy

Janice Bagnall is a 22-year-old post office clerk who has been admitted to the ward for an investigation following a fit at work.

Two days ago, Janice suddenly collapsed at work. Her colleagues reported that she suddenly fell to the floor with a cry, went rigid and then started twitching. She was incontinent of urine.

Janice did not regain consciousness until she was in the ambulance, on the way to hospital. She could remember nothing of what had happened. Janice lives with her boyfriend, Ken, whom she plans to marry next year. They are both anxious about her condition and the outcome of the investigation.

1   State the information needed from Janice on admission in order to plan her care.
2   How could you differentiate between petit mal and grand mal epilepsy for your junior colleague?

The following day after her admission Janice has a grand mal fit while sitting in the day room having coffee with the other patients.

3   Explain the significance of the observations to be made of Janice during this fit.
4   Outline the management of Janice's fit.
5   Describe the role of the nurse in the preparation of Janice for an EEG.
6   What measures should the nurse take to ensure Janice's safety on the ward?

The results of the electroencephalogram and a neurological examination show that Janice has idiopathic epilepsy. She is prescribed oral phenobarbitone 30 mg and phenytoin 100 mg three times a day.

Janice expresses concern that the GPO will no longer want to employ her and that her future with Ken looks bleak.

7   How can you reassure Janice about her job?

8   What should you tell Janice about marriage and having children?
9   What advice should you give Janice and Ken before her discharge home about:
    (a) her condition?
    (b) the prevention of further attacks?
    (c) her drug therapy?
    (d) maintaining a safe environment?
    (e) the management of further fits?

5.1 Answers

1

Information	Use for planning care
Next of kin	Does she want her parents informed?
Knowlege of hospital	Explanations may be needed of routine, ward lay-out, and staff.
Past medical history	Any problems such as diabetes or asthma will need special care
Knowledge of fits	Any misconceptions should be explained.
Usual activities of daily living	This is used to provide a near normal routine, e.g. diet, washing routines.
Problems with activities of daily living	This is used to implement solutions/aids to problems.

2 Ask the junior colleague if she is aware of these two types of epilepsy.

Explain that petit mal epilepsy is characterized by a brief loss of consciousness (5–10 seconds) with minimal or no alterations in muscle tone. It is often mistaken for inattentiveness or daydreaming since behaviour is altered very little. It commonly presents during childhood.

Grand mal epilepsy involves a longer loss of consciousness with generalized muscular contraction and relaxation. Following such a major fit the individual may remain confused for several hours. In a grand mal fit there are four stages:

- **Aura** Fifty per cent of epileptics experience some kind of warning that a fit is going to occur. This aura is an ill-defined sensation which may take the form of a distinctive smell, a flash of light or a feeling of déjà-vu.
- **Tonic phase** During this stage the whole body becomes rigid due to a tonic muscular spasm causing the patient to fall to the ground. As the jaws clamp shut the thoracic and abdominal muscles contract, forcing air through the closed vocal cords. This produces a cry. Laryngospasm and spasm of the chest muscles cause temporary apnoea. This cessation of breathing causes cyanosis.

- **Clonic phase** In this phase the muscles alternately relax and contract, producing jerky movements that involve the patient's whole body. She may salivate and be incontinent.
- **Recovery phase** The patient will sleep for a few minutes or hours. On waking she may complain of a headache or be confused. A minority of patients may experience a period of amnesia or automatic behaviour.

3

Observation	Significance
Janice's activity immediately before the fit	In some individuals emotional stress or a flickering television may induce a fit.
In what part of the body the convulsion started	Symptomatic epilepsy usually causes convulsive movements to start on the opposite side of the body to the cerebral lesion.
Parts of body that were involved	If only one part of the body is affected the epilepsy is likely to be secondary to a cerebral lesion.
Position and movement of the eyes	In focal seizures the eye(s) move away from the side of the cerebral focus.
Skin colour	Janice may need oxygen if she becomes cyanosed.
Respirations	Dyspnoea or stridor may indicate asphyxia.
Time of onset of the fit and duration of each phase	Lengthy phases of muscular contraction or cyanosis may require medical intervention
Any incontinence	Hysterical fits rarely involve incontinence. Janice should be cleaned and dried as soon as possible.
Behaviour after the fit	Janice may need reassurance and close observation if she awakes confused.
Any injuries	A bitten tongue, bruises or grazes may need further attention.

| Total length (in time) of the whole period of fit | Subsequent fits or a close series of fits will indicate status epilepticus. |

4 **DO**:
  - stay with Janice to protect her from injury and observe the fit
  - remove any spectacles or dental plates
  - ensure that she is in no danger (moving furniture if applicable)
  - put a pillow under her head if she is on the floor
  - loosen any tight clothing around the neck which could be pulled tight as the patient jerks around
  - turn her into the recovery position as soon as possible to allow saliva to escape
  - protect her from onlookers (reassuring other patients in the vicinity)
  - allow her to sleep after the fit
  - reassure and reorientate Janice when she awakes and deal with any incontinence
  - observe the characteristics of the fit as above
  - have oxygen and suction available

  DO NOT:
  - restrain her, but guide her movements only to protect her from danger
  - move her unless absolutely necessary
  - try to force anything into her mouth once the tonic stage has commenced in case trauma to the mouth occurs.

5 The nurse should explain to Janice that the initials EEG stand for an electroencephalogram, which is a non-invasive investigation that measures the brain's nerve impulses. She will be asked to wash her hair before the test so that her scalp is clean. Electrodes will be placed on her scalp and she will be left alone, but in sight of the technician. Various stimuli such as flashing lights will be used so that the technician can see if there is any discernible change in the impulses that are recorded on a graph. The test will take about an hour. She will probably want to wash her hair again following the test as the gel used to hold the electrodes in place can be sticky.

6 Although a safe environment for Janice must be ensured, it is also important that her independence is maintained.
  - Use padded cot sides at night and explain the reason for their use to Janice.

- Ask Janice to let you know when she is in the bathroom. Ask her not to lock the door but to use an 'engaged' sign.
- Ensure that she is accompanied if she wants to leave the ward.
- Make sure that the television does not flicker.

7   Epilepsy can be well controlled mostly by medication and should not impair Janice's previous ability to do her job. (Only 15% of epileptics have such uncontrolled epilepsy that they have to be employed in a sheltered workshop.) She should, however, tell her boss of her problem so that someone knows what to do if she should have a fit.

8   Tell Janice that there is no contraindication to marriage but that Ken should be told about the diagnosis. Suggest that they speak to the doctor together so that Ken is fully aware of the situation. It may also help them both to meet another epileptic patient who is well controlled.

There would be no special risks in pregnancy, although she must tell her midwife and obstetrician of her medical history and medication. There is no proof that epilepsy is hereditary.

9   (a) Janice's fits are caused by a spontaneous electrical discharge initiated by a group of over-excitable brain cells. Idiopathic epilepsy means that there is no known reason for these over-excitable cells.

The British Epileptic Society offers literature and practical advice to epileptics and their families.

(b) Janice should be aware of certain factors that may trigger off fits, e.g. flashing disco lights, flickering television, emotional stress or a fever. She may be able to avoid some of these. When she has flu or a sore throat she can take aspirin and cool drinks to bring down her temperature.

(c) It is important that Janice takes her drugs as prescribed if control of her epilepsy is to be successful. She should ensure that she does not run out of tablets. Phenobarbitone can cause excessive drowsiness. Phenytoin can cause a rash, nausea and vomiting, or overgrowth and bleeding of the gums. Janice should report any of these symptoms to her general practitioner. She should visit her general practitioner on a regular basis so that he/she can monitor the effect of the drugs by means of regular blood tests.

She should only drink alcohol in moderation (e.g. one glass of wine at dinner once or twice a week) as alcohol in excess can interfere with the action of her drugs.

Phenytoin should be taken before food to minimize the side-effects of nausea and vomiting.

(d) It must be stressed that Janice can live an almost normal life but that she must not put herself in unnecessary danger in case of a fit. Therefore she should:

- shower rather than bath (if this is not possible a shallow bath is preferable)
- not lock the bathroom door
- not swim or cycle unaccompanied
- not use electric knives, hedge clippers, etc.
- cut her food into small pieces and chew each piece well
- not drive until she has been free of fits during the day for 3 years
- sleep on one firm pillow

(e) If Janice has an aura she should try to get into a safe place and lie down.

Ken should be told what to do in the event of a fit (as in ans. 4).

If Janice has repeated fits without regaining consciousness, which is known as status epilepticus, it can be dangerous. Ken must call an ambulance. He can be reassured that this is rare with good drug treatment.

Ken and Janice should make a record of any fits to report to their general practitioner.

Janice's medication may need to be adjusted.

5.2 Anne Cousins—a woman with meningitis

Anne Cousins is a 28-year-old nursery school teacher. She has been admitted to the ward with a 48-hour history of severe headache, vomiting, hyperpyrexia and neck stiffness. A provisional diagnosis of pyogenic meningitis has been made. She has had a recurrent history of sinusitis.

Anne is married and has twin daughters aged 3 years. Her husband has accompanied her to hospital, leaving the children with a neighbour.

An intravenous infusion is commenced and intravenous penicillin and sulphadiazine have been prescribed to commence after a lumbar puncture has been performed.

1 State, giving reasons, how the nurse should prepare for Mrs Cousins' admission to the ward.
2 How should the nurse assess Mrs Cousins on admission in order to plan her nursing care?
3 What help can Mr Cousins be given with regard to the children?
4 Explain the significance of the observations required to monitor Mrs Cousins' condition.
5 Describe how Mrs Cousins' headache may be relieved.

Later in the day Mrs Cousins' husband comes to speak to you. He asks you to explain his wife's condition and wants to know if it is infectious. Will she have any brain damage as a result of the condition?

6 How should you respond to Mr Cousins' enquiries?
7 How should the nurse prepare Mrs Cousins for her lumbar puncture?
8 How might the nurse relieve Mrs Cousins' anxieties about her children?
9 Briefly describe the role of the nurse in the administration of intravenous antibiotics.
10 What advice should the nurse give to Mr and Mrs Cousins when Mrs Cousins is ready for discharge from hospital?

5.2   Answers

1

Preparation	Reason
Side room	This allows for a quiet environment.
Window blinds drawn	This relieves photophobia.
One pillow	Mrs Cousins will need to lie flat due to neck stiffness.
Vomit bowl and tissues discreetly available	Vomiting is a common feature of meningitis.

From Mrs Cousins' history, the most likely cause of her meningitis is a streptococcal infection. However, it may be hospital policy to isolate her until meningococcal meningitis is positively ruled out.

2   Mrs Cousins should be settled comfortably and then her husband should be asked for most of the details of the nursing assessment to allow her to rest.

Before leaving her, the nurse should make an initial assessment by:

- **observing the state of her mouth** Is it very dry? Does her breath smell? Are her lips dry or cracked?
- **taking her temperature** Does she feel hot? Is she sweating?
- **observing her manner** Does she wince when moved? Does her facial expression reveal pain? Does she seem irritable when disturbed?
- **observing her level of consciousness** Does she seem fully alert or drowsy?

The nurse should then ask Mr Cousins the following questions:

- How will he manage with the children?
- Has she been vomiting? Has she been able to eat or drink?
- Does he have any special worries?
- Did she have any other problems at home relating to this illness or to any other medical problem?

3   As Mrs Cousins works there may be some arrangements to care for the children already. Discuss how these could be extended to meet hospitalization. Enquire if there is a relative who could be contacted to come and look after them.

If these options are not possible inform the medical social worker who could organize a home help, a registered child minder, or residential nursery places, depending on Mr Cousins' needs.

4

Observation	Significance
4-hourly blood pressure, pulse and respirations	Hypertension, bradycardia and respiratory distress indicate pressure on the medulla from raised intracranial pressure due to cerebral oedema or abscess formation.
1-hourly temperature	Continued hyperpyrexia indicates pressure on the hypothalamus from raised intracranial pressure. Observation of the temperature also monitors the degree of pyrexia, the effect of reducing methods, and ensures that the temperature is not lowered too quickly.
4-hourly level of consciousness	Increasing coma indicates cerebral dysfunction due to raised pressure.
Any twitching or fitting	Such features are indicative of cerebral oedema.
Fluid intake and output	Hyperpyrexia and vomiting may lead to dehydration. Observation of the fluid intake and output also monitors the degree of vomiting.
Any visual or hearing loss	Severe inflammation and cerebral oedema can damage the auditory or optic nerves.
Pupil size	It is unnecessary to test pupil reaction to light in a photophobic patient but pupil size can be observed for inequality and dilatation, which is a sign of raised intercranial pressure.

5
- Provide analgesia, e.g. codeine phosphate 30–60 mg, 4–6 hourly or intramuscularly.
- Lie her down in a quiet, dark side room.
- Restrict visitors to husband and close relatives (e.g. Mrs Cousins' mother). Explain to them that they should sit quietly with Mrs Cousins.
- Plan the nursing care so that disturbance is minimal.
- Prevent coughing and straining at stool, which will aggra-

vate a headache. Encourage deep breathing exercises to prevent chest infection. Administer a daily aperient, e.g. Dorbanex 10 ml.

- Lie her flat with one pillow.

6   Explain to Mr Cousins that meningitis is inflammation of the meninges, the three membranes that cover the brain and spinal cord. It is most likely in Mrs Cousins' case that the infection reached the meninges via her infected sinuses. The inflamed meninges irritate the brain itself and cause Mrs Cousins' problems. This type of meningeal infection can be treated with antibiotics and is not infectious. With prompt treatment there are no long-term complications.

Ask him if he has any other questions.

7   Explain meningitis as above. Explain that positive identification of the causative organism is needed to ensure that the correct antibiotic is used. To do this a specimen of cerebral spinal fluid is needed. This fluid flows between the meninges and will carry the organism.

Mrs Cousins will need to curl up in a ball with her spine along the edge of the bed. A nurse will be with her all the time. The doctor will inject a local anaesthetic into her spine. This may sting momentarily. Then all she will feel is pressure on her spine as a specimen is withdrawn via a needle and syringe. A small dressing will be put over this injection site.

8   Talk to Mr Cousins. Ask him to relay messages back and forth to his wife. Perhaps the children could draw pictures for their mother. Let Mrs Cousins use the trolley telephone to talk to the twins.

Find out whether photographs of the twins can be brought in to the ward.

Arrange for the person looking after the twins to visit briefly to reassure Mrs Cousins that all is well.

9   The administration of intravenous drugs is considered part of the extended role of the nurse (i.e. it is not considered part of the basic role of the nurse and is not taught during nurse training).

The nurse administering intravenous drugs must therefore be a registered nurse. She must also have completed a recognized programme of preparation and received a Certificate of Competence according to hospital policy. She must also agree to undertake the procedure; if she is at all doubtful about the situation, the delegating doctor should be asked to perform the task. The doctor should always be present for the first intravenous injection in case of adverse reaction.

Tasks such as intravenous injections should not take priority over nursing care. If there is a heavy workload of nursing care the extended role should be performed by the doctor.

It is also important that the nurse keeps up-to-date and should have an opportunity to review her knowledge of the extended role annually.

Before giving any intravenous drugs the nurse should be familiar with the drug, its action and expected effect, as well as possible side-effects.

10 Warn the couple that it will probably be at least 3 months before Mrs Cousins feels well enough to resume normal activities. She should not worry about this but should plan periods of rest throughout the day. She will need help with the twins as well as with the housework. The medical social worker will be able to arrange this help if necessary.

5.3   Mrs Frost—a woman with multiple sclerosis

Rebecca Frost has had multiple sclerosis for 10 years. She is now 34 years old and has been admitted to the ward with an exacerbation of her condition. This regression has resulted in a paralysis of both legs. Up until this admission she had weakness of her legs but was able to walk with the aid of sticks. She has had an indwelling catheter for the last 2 years.

She is married with three children—David aged 12, Sarah aged 10 and Andrew aged 7.

Injections of adrenocorticotrophic hormone injections have been prescribed.

1   How would you explain to a junior colleague:
   (a) Mrs Frost's condition?
   (b) the purpose of her drug therapy?
2   Mr Frost says that he wants to plan for the future and asks you to describe the course of his wife's condition. What should you say?
3   Plan the care needed to monitor Mrs Frost for any potential problems of her drug therapy.
4   Describe the complications of long-term catheters. Explain how these can be prevented.
5   How can Mrs Frost's family be taught to care for her at home?
6   Discuss Mr Frost's possible problems.
7   Mr Frost asks you how he should deal with his wife's mood swings. How can you reply?
8   What advice should the nurse give Mrs Frost about avoiding future exacerbations?
9   Describe the help available in the community to help the Frost family.

5.3 Answers

1 (a) Multiple sclerosis is a chronic, progressive, disabling condition of the nervous system. Its cause is unknown but various theories are at present being researched such as allergic reactions, viral infections or a chemical or enzyme disturbance.

The features of multiple sclerosis are due to a breakdown of the myelin sheath which surrounds the axon of nerve fibres. The functions of myelin are to act as insulation and to speed up the transmission of nerve impulses. The demyelination that occurs in multiple sclerosis is of patchy distribution, so individuals have varying features depending on the area of the nervous system affected.

In the early stages of the disease, healing of the affected area may occur to some extent, and function of the part may return either partially or completely. But with each episode the features tend to be more severe and last longer, and the disability may become permanent with degeneration of the axons themselves.

These periods of remission and exacerbation are a characteristic pattern of multiple sclerosis.

(b) Adrenocorticotrophic hormone (ACTH) is an adrenal steroid which is used for its anti-inflammatory action. It is thought that ACTH, used in the acute phase of an exacerbation, can reduce the inflammation of the nerve fibre caused by the disease process. By reducing inflammation the exacerbation and any permanent disability should be lessened.

2 The prognosis for multiple sclerosis is very variable. Although some patients experience gradual deterioration, this is not invariably so. Patients do not die from multiple sclerosis and can live for an average life-span.

Because the characteristics of the condition are periods of remission and exacerbation, it is impossible to foretell a precise pattern of events.

However, from Mrs Frost's history it seems likely that she may eventually need a wheel-chair. The nursing staff and social workers can help to overcome the problems this eventuality may cause.

3

Potential problem	Care
Hypertension due to sodium and water retention	• Daily blood pressure measurement • Fluid balance chart • Weekly weight measurement
Steroid-induced diabetes	• Urine test on alternate days for glucose
Infection due to increased susceptibility	• 4-hourly temperature measurement. (Minor changes will not be apparent, so the nurse should observe for other signs of infection, e.g. infected urine.)

4

Complication	Prevention
Infection via: • trauma of catheter at urethral orifice	Attach catheter to patient's leg with adhesive tape to prevent pull.
• contaminants around urethral orifice	Use a shower rather than a bath. Clean catheter exit site and genitalia at least daily.
• connection between catheter and drainage tubing	Do not break connection unless changing drainage bag. Use a sample sleeve to take specimens.
• outlet tap of drainage bag	Ensure that hands are washed before emptying bag into clean, dry jug. Do not allow bag to drag along floor.

• reflux of urine	Ensure drainage bag and tubing are always below the level of the patient's bladder.
	    Ensure tubing does not become kinked or compressed.
	    Because ascending infection can lead to

	pyelonephritis, observe urine for infection (sediment, pus, smell, colour) daily. Take at least weekly specimens. Encourage high output by advising patient to drink 2–3 litres per day.
• catheter itself acting as a foreign body	Use silastic catheters for long-term use. Change every 4–6 weeks.
Pain due to bladder spasm	Use size 18–20 Foley catheter. If pain troublesome a muscle relaxant can be prescribed (e.g. Baclofen).

5   The family can be involved in her care while she is in hospital.

Mr Frost can be taught, with his eldest son, how to lift his wife safely. They can also be shown how to help her to move from the bed to the chair.

Mr Frost can be shown how to care for his wife's pressure areas, catheter care, passive limb exercises and correct positioning of the paralysed limbs. By working alongside the nurses, he can build up his confidence in these skills and gradually take over by himself.

6   The psychological and social problems for Mr Frost may be great.

He will be worried about seeing his wife deteriorate and become more disabled. He may be concerned about how he will cope physically and mentally with her dependence.

He may not be used to helping in the home and may not know how to take over the housework and cooking.

He may be anxious about the children's reactions to a 'crippled' mother.

He may worry about leaving his wife alone while he is at work and the children are at school.

He may think that sexual intercourse with his wife is no longer possible or he may even find her disability unattractive.

If the marriage is already unsteady, he may be thinking of divorce but could think it is his duty to then stay with the family.

7   Mood swings are common among patients with multiple sclerosis. This may be for two reasons. First, it may be due to damage to the central nervous system in the area that controls emotion; secondly, it may be caused by deep anx-

iety about her illness, disability and prognosis. Both will contribute to alternating euphoria and depression.

If crying is a reaction to concern and fear about her condition, Mr Frost should try and take time to allow her to express these anxieties so that they can talk together about the problem. If, however, Mrs Frost is crying for no apparent reason, even to herself, the episode should be accepted as a feature of the illness.

8   Mrs Frost should be advised not to become overtired as excessive fatigue can cause an exacerbation. Any late nights should be counteracted by an afternoon rest beforehand or a day of restful activities afterwards.

She should try to avoid infections by avoiding close contact with friends who have colds or influenza. Urinary tract infections should be avoided as stated in ans. **4**. To ensure that her resistance to infection is good, she should eat a well-balanced diet. She should continue with deep breathing exercises at home to avoid a chest infection due to her relative immobility.

She should also try to avoid stressful situations. Deep breathing exercises may be helpful in avoiding stress.

9   • **Multiple Sclerosis Society** This provides support and information for patients and their families, and organizes outings.

• **Community nurse** He/she can visit to help with bathing and changing the catheter.

• **Home help** He/she will help with heavy housework and shopping if necessary.

• **Aids for the handicapped** The occupational therapist and physiotherapist can assess the home for alterations/aids needed. This work can be organized by the social services department.

• **Social worker** He/she can advise on supplementary benefits if needed. Mr Frost may be entitled to an attendance allowance if Mrs Frost requires continuous care throughout the day and night.

5.4 Mr Jackson—who has had a subarachnoid haemorrhage

Mr Dennis Jackson, aged 42 years, has been admitted to your ward following a subarachnoid haemorrhage. He has had a 12-hour history of an increasingly severe headache, associated with vomiting, visual disturbances and increasing drowsiness. His wife says that he has been complaining of a headache for the last week. On admission, Mr Jackson is conscious but drowsy.

Mr Jackson is a self-employed driving instructor. He has two children, aged 12 and 14 years.

1 How could Mr Jackson's condition be explained to a junior colleague?
2 Describe the potential problems specific to Mr Jackson. How may these be prevented?
3 Explain the role of the nurse in the preparation of Mr Jackson for a CAT scan.
4 How should the following be explained to a junior nurse:
   (a) the purpose of a lumbar puncture in this situation?
   (b) the role of the nurse before, during and after Mr Jackson's lumbar puncture?

It is decided to treat Mr Jackson conservatively. It is explained to him and his wife that this will involve up to 3 weeks of strict bed rest, followed by a period of remobilization and convalescence.

5 Mrs Jackson asks you why surgery has not been considered viable. How should you reply?
6 Mrs Jackson asks how she can reassure her children about their father. What advice can be given?
7 Describe how Mr Jackson may be protected from developing complications of immobility.
8 Explain how Mr Jackson should be remobilized after his period of bed rest.

5.4   Answers

1   First, check the junior colleague's present level of know-
    ledge. This could be done by asking her to draw a diagram
    of the meninges indicating the area of the haemorrhage.

    Confirm that a subarachnoid haemorrhage is bleeding
    into the subarachnoid space, i.e. between the arachnoid and
    the pia mater.

    The bleeding may be caused by a head injury (rare),
    following neurosurgery or, most commonly, by the rupture
    of an abnormal blood vessel in the subarachnoid space.
    The abnormal blood vessel may be an angioma (a mass of
    abnormal fragile blood vessels) or an aneurysm (a localized
    dilatation of an artery which ruptures due to a congenital
    weakness and/or the effect of degenerative processes).

    Bleeding into a confined space causes features of raised
    intracranial pressure as the build-up of blood presses onto
    the cerebral cortex.

2

Potential problem	Preventive care
Coning (herniation of the lower portion of the brain stem or medulla through the foramen magnum) due to increasing intracranial pressure	Make 1-hourly neurological observations to monitor the degree of raised intracranial pressure. Check: • level of consciousness • pupil size • pupil reaction to light • blood pressure • pulse • respirations • temperature • motor function
Re-bleeding from the original site may occur if the blood pressure is allowed to rise.	Keep blood pressure stable by: • bed rest with one pillow • advising the patient to try to avoid coughing and sneezing • preventing constipation by daily laxatives (e.g. Dorbanex) Encourage clotting by:

- administering the prescribed fibrinolytic (e.g. aminocaproic acid)

Ensure that the patient is calm by:
- explanations
- reassurances
- limited visitors only
- analgesia (e.g. codeine phosphate)

Vasospasm may occur in the damaged vessels, leading to ischaemia and infarction of the cerebral tissue.

Keep the patient at rest mentally and physically as above, and avoid antihypertensive drugs.

3 The investigation should first be explained to the patient. CAT stands for 'computed axial tomography'. It is very much like an X-ray. The patient will lie on a table with his head inside a large, helmet-like camera. This will rotate to take a picture of his brain from all different angles. It is quite painless. The computer then produces pictures of the information that has been scanned. The results should be available immediately.

The nurse should stay with Mr Jackson in view of his serious condition to ensure that he does not deteriorate during the scan, which takes only a few minutes. The scan will identify the site of the bleeding.

4 (a) First, check that the junior nurse understands what is meant by a lumbar pucture.

Confirm that the bleeding in this situation is in the subarachnoid space. A specimen of cerebrospinal fluid will therefore show blood if a subarachnoid haemorrhage has occurred. The presence of blood will be equal throughout the three specimens.

The presence of blood after a subarachnoid haemorrhage may not be obvious; old blood may appear as a yellow colouring of the cerebrospinal fluid, and is called xanthochromia.

(b) The nurse's responsibilities include an explanation to the patient (according to his level of understanding) of the need to appreciate that a small amount of cerebrospinal fluid will be removed from his back. This is achieved by a special needle inserted into the lumbar region of his back.

A local anaesthetic is injected into this area first, so no pain should be felt. He will need to lie still.

The nurse should position the patient on his side with his knees drawn up. His head and shoulders should be bent forward so that his spine is flexed. His back should be at the edge of the bed. The nurse should stay at the patient's head to reassure him and observe for any distress.

The nurse should set up the trolley aseptically. She should check that the specimen bottles are labelled 1, 2 and 3 and that they are sent to the laboratory.

Following the procedure the patient should continue to lie flat to prevent coning. Any worsening of his headache may be a sign of coning and should be reported immediately.

5 Explain carefully to Mrs Jackson that there may be two reasons why surgery has not been considered:

1 Surgery will only be performed if bleeding is continuing and causing pressure on the brain tissue.

2 The site and/or size of the bleeding vessel may be inaccessible, involving too much damage to vital structures within the brain.

Also explain that surgery does not invariably result in total cure. It holds considerable risks and the patient can be left with a degree of dysfunction afterwards.

6 Mrs Jackson can only be given suggestions about how to handle this problem.

She should explain Mr Jackson's condition to the children so that they can appreciate why he is so ill. (Explain it first to Mrs Jackson using diagrams that she can take home, so that the children can then appreciate his headache and drowsiness and the need for a quiet environment.)

They should be allowed to see their father and, after the above explanations, should appreciate the need for short, calm visits.

They should not be excluded from their mother's feelings. She should try to express her fears to them so that they can appreciate her needs.

They should be given responsibilities so that they do not feel forgotten in this time of stress.

They could express their feelings for their father by writing to him or making him things.

Mrs Jackson should also find time for them to express their fears without feeling that they are imposing on her stress.

Mrs Jackson will mostly be concerned that her husband may die and about how she will cope.

As Mr Jackson is self-employed, money may be a worry as he will be in hospital for some time.

She will be anxious about the children and possibly she will feel torn between being with them or her husband.

She may be concerned about a reversal of roles, now that she is head of the household.

She may worry about her husband having a permanent disability and how she will cope with this.

7

Complication	Care
Boredom	• Arrange a bed by the window with a view. • When able, organize books with a stand, and television. Provide him with jobs (filling in charts, etc.). • Arrange for an occupational therapist to visit.
Chest infection	• Encourage breathing exercises.
Pressure sores	• Keep the skin clean and dry. • Change his position 2-hourly.
Deep vein thrombosis	• Encourage leg exercises when able (passive exercises before this) and the use of thromboembolic deterrent (TED) stockings.
Urinary problems	• Ensure that the bottle is always within reach • Observe the urine output and the characteristics of the urine. • Report any drop in output or signs of infection immediately.
Constipation	• Encourage fresh fruit and bran with cereal. • Give Dorbanex 10 ml every evening. • Ensure privacy when a bedpan is needed. • Encourage regular bowel habits.

| Indigestion/ anorexia | • Offer small, easily digestible foods.
• Ensure that the meals are attractive.
• Serve his favourite foods.
• Ask his wife to bring in treats. |

8   Mr Jackson should be remobilized very gradually.

After a period of 2–3 weeks, if he is asymptomatic, he should initially be given an extra pillow over the following week to slowly raise him to a sitting position.

When he has achieved this he can sit out in a chair. This should only be for short periods for the first 2–3 days. Once he is able to sit up he can also use the commode.

Once he is able to sit in the chair for 2–3 hours, he can start to stand and walk for short distances out to the toilet at first.

Two weeks after the end of his bed rest he should be ready to go home but should be instructed to continue to increase his activity on a gradual basis.

He should be warned to avoid anything that would increase intracranial pressure, e.g. extreme stress, constipation, chronic coughing/sneezing.

Further Reading

General nursing

Brunner, L. & Suddarth, D. (1982) *The Lippincott Manual of Medical–Surgical Nursing*, Vol. 1–3. London: Harper & Row.

Clark, J.E., Sage, C.A. & Attree, M.J. (1985) *Revise Essential Nursing Care*, Letts Study Aids. London: Charles Letts & Co.

Faulkner, A. (1985) *Nursing—A Creative Approach*. London: Baillière Tindall.

Hunt, P. & Sendell, B. (1984) *Nursing the Adult with a Specific Physiological Disturbance*. London: The Macmillan Press.

Lewer, H. & Robertson, L. (1983) *Care of the Child*. London: The Macmillan Press.

Long, B.C. & Phipps, W.J. (1985) *Essentials of Medical–Surgical Nursing*. St Louis: C.V. Mosby.

Parkin, D. (1985) *Revise Nursing RGN*, Letts Study Aids. London: Charles Letts & Co.

Roper, N., Logan, W. & Tierney, A. (1985) *The Elements of Nursing*. Edinburgh: Churchill Livingstone.

The Royal Marsden Hospital (1984) In Pritchard, A. & Walker, V.A. (eds.) *Manual of Clinical Nursing Policies and Procedures*. London: Harper & Row.

Specific to topics included in this book

Hamilton, H. & Rose, M.B. (1984) *Respiratory Disorders*. Pennsylvania: Springhouse Corporation.

Lewer, H. & Robertson, L. (1983) *Care of the Child*. London: The Macmillan Press.

O'Brien, D.A. & Shirley, A. (1985) *High Dependency Nursing Care*. Edinburgh: Churchill Livingstone.

Robinson, J. (1979) *Coping with Neurological Problems Proficiently*. Pennsylvania: Intermed Communications Inc.

Robinson, J. (1979) *Using Crisis Intervention Wisely*. Pennsylvania: Intermed Communications Inc.

Wells, B. (1983) *Body and Personality*. London: Longman Group.